Acknowledgements

This research has its origins as a project funded by the National Children's Office Research Programme. It was undertaken in 2005 at the Faculty of Law, University College Cork, by project leader Dr. Ursula Kilkelly, together with Mary Donnelly and Dr. Deirdre Madden. The research assistants were Anne O'Reilly and Sylvia Hoare. We would like to thank Anne, Sylvia and Deirdre for their considerable contribution to the research and we are also extremely grateful to Dr. Siobhán McAllister of Queen's University Belfast for her assistance in planning the interviews with the children.

The assistance of many NGOs was vital in the completion of this research. We are particularly grateful to Mary O'Connor, Chief Executive, Children in Hospital Ireland, who assisted with the planning process, and to the following people and organisations who were involved directly or indirectly in the research: Heart Children Ireland; TCCUP; ISPCC; Traveller Visibility Group; Longford Traveller Movement; Coeliac Society of Ireland; Barretstown Castle; Wesley Crawford; Brainwave (Irish Epilepsy Association); and Enable Ireland.

Others provided invaluable support by sharing literature and ideas on our research and commenting on earlier drafts. Special thanks are due to Mary Godfrey, Department of Health and Children; Veronica Lambert, Trinity College Dublin; and Eileen Savage, University College Cork. We would also like to acknowledge the assistance of Professor Colin Bradley, Head of the Department of General Practice, University College Cork. Thank you to Sinead Hanafin and her colleagues in the Office of the Minister for Children for their support in bringing the research to publication.

Finally, our gratitude is due to all the people — children, parents and health professionals — who shared their experiences and perspectives with us. We hope this report adequately acknowledges the immense contribution they made to our understanding of the issues at the heart of this research.

Ursula Kilkelly and Mary Donnelly

EXECUTIVE SUMMARY

Under Article 12 of the United Nations Convention on the Rights of the Child (UNCRC), every child has the right to express his or her views on all matters affecting him or her and to have these views given due weight in accordance with the child's age and maturity. The duty to listen to children is thus a legal one, although facilitating the participation of children in decisions concerning them has many social, political and, in the case of healthcare, therapeutic advantages.

To date, attention has focused on ways to involve children in a meaningful way in the areas of policy development and governance in both the statutory and voluntary sectors. Little has been done to identify whether children are involved in decision-making in the private sector and to develop models of communication appropriate to this area.

This research aims to fill this gap by exploring the extent to which children are listened to in the healthcare setting. It does so by:
• recording the experiences and attitudes of children, parents and health professionals; and
• auditing the training and educational materials of health professionals.

It explains best practice in the area of participation with children in the healthcare setting, identifies barriers to implementing this best practice and makes recommendations as to how the best practice that does exist can be developed and mainstreamed throughout the healthcare environment.

This research examined within a legal framework the extent to which children's voices are being heard in the healthcare setting. Its key strength is the combination of a range of stakeholder perspectives combined with a curriculum audit to advance a unique and focused understanding of the issue addressed.

The experiences and attitudes of 52 children, 30 parents and 50 health professionals were gathered via group and individual interviews. The research also undertook an audit of the education and teaching curricula of a range of health professionals. Due to the short time-frame of the research and its objective to take a 'snapshot' of children's experiences, convenience sampling was used to identify participants. Thus, it is not possible to say the extent to which these views are representative of children, parents and health professionals as a whole.

Findings

Views of children
The children interviewed for this research varied in age, gender, background and the level of contact they had had with the healthcare system. Yet, despite these variables they consistently identified the importance of being heard by health professionals and routinely explained the importance to them of being provided with age-appropriate explanations and information to help them cope with the consultation and treatment process. They articulated clearly a need to be understood and to be treated with empathy, kindness and good humour during illness, whether serious or not so serious. The children interviewed identified a range of both practical and principled reasons as to why this was the case.

Interviews with children showed a variation in the extent to which their preferred model of participation matched the reality of their experience. While more extensive research is required before definitive conclusions can be reached, it appears from this research at least that children who have come into contact with specialists in children's health or those working in children's hospitals had more favourable experiences in this regard in that they were better informed and more involved in their healthcare decisions.

Children also made valuable suggestions on how their interactions with health professionals could be improved. While many of the children referred specifically to their doctor in this regard, their recommendations — that training be undertaken with regard to effective communication with children and age-appropriate language and props be used — were directed at *all* health professionals. Furthermore, their recommendations that waiting areas and hospitals be made more child-friendly, particularly for older children, are simple yet clearly important to improve the quality of the healthcare experience for all children. All of these findings are consistent with research carried out elsewhere.

Views of parents

A diverse group of parents was interviewed, including some who were parents of the children interviewed. Their views on their experiences of attending health professionals with their children were rich and varied. It is perhaps simplistic to conclude that the views of those with a high level of contact with the healthcare system (such as those whose children have long-term and serious health problems) show a greater awareness of the importance of their child's participation in the consultation and treatment processes. However, on the basis of interviews with parents, greater involvement with the health professional seems to impact on parental views on participation, together with other factors such as the fact that a child undergoing long-term treatment will develop and mature throughout this process.

More generally, a range of factors affects parents' views of the child's capacity and readiness to be fully involved in any communication with health professionals, not least the parents' own understanding of the process and of the right of their child to participate in it. An important issue identified in the interviews, and confirmed by previous research, is the conflict that can arise between the parent and the health professional regarding the process of consulting and informing the child about their health and healthcare. It was found that parents who did not appreciate health professionals' attempts to involve their child directly in the process were motivated by a variety of reasons, ranging from a lack of awareness of the child's need and right to be involved, to the need to protect the child from unnecessary anxiety. This demonstrates the complexity of this issue. It also highlights the importance of raising awareness about the child's right to be heard among parents and the need to ensure that health professionals receive the necessary skills and training on how to communicate with both parents and children in the healthcare setting.

At the same time, parents' identification of the need to adapt the hospital environment for children is entirely consistent with children's own views, as is their recommendation that health professionals need to show greater empathy with their child patients, to build relations with them based on trust and to communicate more directly with them. The need to provide training for health professionals in this area is also entirely consistent with the recommendation of children and health professionals themselves. This is one area where unanimity was found to exist between all interviewees.

Views of health professionals

Many of the issues raised by health professionals were already identified in the interviews with children or parents, showing a consistency in the research carried out and the shared experiences and perspectives of all parties involved in children's health. The influential role of factors such as the personality and attitude of the health professional, the lack of training in communication skills and limited resources such as time and physical environment are all themes that resonate throughout this research. These barriers to participation have also been clearly identified in previous research of this kind.

The research found a clear difference between the approaches of some professionals, particularly those with specialist training in children's healthcare and those who have specialised in other areas but nonetheless treat children. In addition to the need to address the training of all health professionals in this context, this also raises the need to adopt a common and a multidisciplinary approach to communicating with children throughout the healthcare system. The different demands and challenges faced by health professionals must, however, be taken into account since all have different roles within the system, as well as different time and resources at their disposal.

Although the duty to listen to children is clearly placed on the shoulders of the health professional, interviews with the professionals themselves confirm that the role of parents in the process is as influential in practice as in theory. Indeed, consistent with other research, interviews with health professionals confirm that the dynamic between them and parents is a hugely significant factor in how they communicate with their child patients. The fact that, for many health professionals, parents' influence on the effectiveness of communication with children is decisive in either positive or negative terms means that any training of health professionals on listening to children must also address these tensions and how to deal with them.

Education and curriculum review

No single conclusion can be drawn regarding the extent to which the training of health professionals on communication with children meets the demands of Article 12 of the UN Convention on the Rights of the Child. According to this research, there is a notable difference between the education and training of nurses and therapists, on the one hand, and that of the medical and dentistry professions on the other. While clinical medical education, which is currently largely undocumented, may indeed incorporate the practice of communicating with children, the current lack of documentation made this difficult to measure. Moreover, improvements and changes to curricula in the medical profession in particular are ongoing and may bring about further developments in this area in the near future.

The nursing profession and others, including occupational therapists and speech and language therapists, appear to have made greater progress in the incorporation into their educational programmes of theoretical and practical approaches to listening to children. While at an early stage of development, best practice nonetheless appears to exist in the education and training of these professions, which have integrated communicating with children into their educational programmes in a formal manner. In contrast, analysis of educational curricula for the medical profession indicates a lack of detailed or structured focus on either the theoretical or practical framework within which the voice of the child can effectively be heard in the healthcare setting. To date, the medical profession appears to have made more modest progress towards the incorporation of communication skills into education and training curricula, and has developed very limited, if any, training programmes on communicating with children.

Interviews with health professionals confirm the lacuna in their training in this regard, as well as the lack of guidance from their professional bodies on the topic. Many health professionals who had not experienced any training on communicating with children had developed their own methodologies through emulation of senior colleagues, on-the-job training and reflection on specific case histories with clinical colleagues. Those who had experienced training took a more structured and perhaps formalised approach in their communication with children.

In light of the mixed progress towards incorporating communicating with children into the education and training curricula of health professionals, it is important that awareness of the need for such training is on the increase. The current state of change of the medical curriculum in particular means that the time is opportune for cooperation within the healthcare setting on this issue. While different approaches will be required in different areas, considerable good practice, which is equally relevant and appropriate to all professions, can be shared widely. The mainstreaming of theoretical and practical knowledge as to how to communicate effectively with children is to be strongly encouraged.

In addition to developing competencies in this area, however, a broader issue arises with regard to the need to raise awareness of children's rights among all health professionals and the need to establish a common understanding of the importance and value of respecting the right of children to be heard. In this regard, training and education for health professionals must aim to develop both the skills to communicate effectively with children and the attitude and mind-set necessary to achieve greater respect for their rights in practice. The need to incorporate such training into the education of health professionals, as well as to integrate it into continuing professional development programmes, is evident from this research. Its clear relationship to the clinical skills so important to all health professionals may help to convince already stretched practitioners of the importance of undertaking such training.

Best practice in communicating with children

Best practice regarding communication with children can be summarised as follows:
- The child must be involved in treatment decisions as far as possible, bearing in mind his/her capacity to understand and willingness to be involved.
- The patient's parents or carers must be involved in treatment decisions.
- The views of children must be sought and taken into account.

- The relationship between health professional and child should be based on truthfulness, clarity and awareness of the child's age and maturity.
- Children must be listened to and their questions responded to, clearly and truthfully.
- Communication with children must be an ongoing process.
- Training in communication skills with children is an essential component of appropriate professional education.

In this research, children, parents and health professionals identified a wide range of approaches for listening to children in the healthcare setting. Regardless of their different perspectives, there was a remarkable degree of consistency between the models favourably identified in this context and the best practice identified above, although some parents were critical about professionals who, they believed, marginalised them from the process.

Best practice was found throughout the healthcare system among specialists in children's health and non-specialists, in both general and specialist children's hospitals and in the community. While positive initiatives were identified in all areas of the healthcare profession examined, positive experiences were more likely among those who had been trained in children's health and/or those who worked in a specialist environment (unit or hospital) for children.

The positive initiatives shown by health professionals can be summarised as follows:
- Addressing children directly during the consultation process (e.g. by asking them personally about their ailment or condition). This is important regardless of the child's age, although the level of complexity, amount of information imparted and involvement of children in any decision-making process should be appropriate to the child's age and maturity. Although this will depend on the setting, efforts to communicate directly with children should not exclude parents and vice versa.
- Adopting an age-appropriate approach to treating children, which takes into account their development and capacity to understand.
- Chatting with the child to make him or her feel relaxed, while also respecting personal boundaries.
- Preparing children adequately for what is about to happen in a treatment or procedure, and giving them the opportunity to ask questions and to prepare themselves.
- Empathising with children, being light-hearted and good-humoured where appropriate.
- Using age-appropriate language and props to explain things to children, including their condition, the prescribed treatment or the procedure about to be undertaken.
- Giving children choices as to how they want to proceed.
- Being honest with children in order to build a relationship of trust.
- Creating an environment in which children are encouraged to ask questions.
- Making the healthcare environment, including waiting rooms and treatment areas, child-friendly for children of all ages.

Obstacles to communicating with children
Similar to the findings on the subject of best practice *(see above)*, the research also identified, with remarkable consistency, the obstacles that currently prevent children being listened to in the healthcare setting. While some of these barriers are attitudinal and will require time and effort to break down, others are structural and could be addressed with the appropriate use of resources. Some are within the gift of the health professionals themselves, while others fall under the responsibility of the Department of Health and Children. These barriers to communication include:
- **Training and experience:** While children's specialists appear to be aware of and practise best practice regarding communicating with children, few non-specialists have received adequate training or education on children's rights, child development or ways of listening effectively to children in the healthcare setting. On-the-job training is not always an appropriate or effective way of providing this experience and has limitations that must be recognised in this context.
- **Intervention of parents:** The attitude and approach of parents can play both a negative and a positive role in the relationship between their child and the health professional, and can be decisive as to whether children are listened to in the healthcare setting.

- **Time:** The limited time available for consultations means that professionals do not have as long as they might need to ensure children are heard during the consultation and treatment process.
- **Physical environment:** The lack of available and appropriate space hinders effective communication between health professionals and their child patients.
- **Personality of the health professional:** The personality or attitude of individual health professionals often plays a significant role as to whether or not they listen to children.

Recommendations

The following recommendations are made with a view to addressing the obstacles and challenges that currently exist to listening to children in the healthcare setting:

1. **Public information campaign:** A public information campaign aimed at children and adults needs to take place to raise awareness of the right of the child to be heard.
2. **Training:** Child development, children's rights and appropriate ways to communicate with children of all ages and stages of development should be incorporated into the training of all health professionals. This should also address the role of parents in this process.
3. **Protocols and best practice:** Protocols need to be developed between all health professionals, establishing best practice and shared approaches to communicating with children.
4. **Research:** Further research should be undertaken into the extent to which children are listened to in the healthcare setting. In particular, the experiences of teenagers and children and young people with disabilities should be taken into account.

1 INTRODUCTION TO CHILDREN'S PARTICIPATION RIGHTS

Article 12 of the United Nations Convention on the Rights of the Child (UNCRC) guarantees to every child capable of forming his or her views the right to express those views freely in all matters affecting him or her. It also recognises the right of the child to have those views given due weight in accordance with the child's age and maturity. Together, these represent the right of the child to be heard and to participate in decisions made concerning him or her.

Article 12 places a legally binding duty on all States that have ratified the UNCRC, including Ireland. Its implementation also represents a moral imperative for adults to respect children as autonomous beings and rights-holders, and to promote and vindicate their right to be heard in all decisions taken concerning them.

Importance of participation for children

At the same time that the child's right to be heard and to participate in decisions made about them achieved recognition in international law, the growing influence of the consumer and an increased understanding of children as competent social actors together promoted increased acceptance of the importance of participation with children (Sinclair, 2004). As well as being a legal right and duty, therefore, facilitating the participation of children in decision-making is important for political and social reasons insofar as it improves services, decision-making and broader democratic processes; promotes children's protection and enhances their skills; and empowers and enhances children's self-esteem (Sinclair, 2004; Lansdown, 2001).

While little is known about the outcomes of the involvement and participation of children in decisions about their own healthcare, there is evidence that it may have a positive effect on the outcome of healthcare treatment. In particular, increased child involvement in healthcare decisions has been shown to increase adherence, adaptation, sense of competence and understanding of their illness (Angst and Deatrick, 1996). Moreover, the way adolescents are treated by health professionals has been shown to be an important predictor of their satisfaction with healthcare (Beresford and Sloper, 2003). Conversely, early and independent control of treatment decisions has been shown to result in poorer health outcomes and may be associated with children feeling depressed, isolated and abandoned (Angst and Deatrick, 1996; Law Reform Committee, 2006).

There is also a therapeutic argument favouring the provision of information. A body of empirical research on informed consent indicates that patients who have been involved with their healthcare decisions, including having more full information, tend to respond better to treatment (Fallowfield et al, 1990). To date, this work has for the main part been concerned with adults. However, it would seem that children and young people may also experience benefits from greater levels of involvement in their healthcare decisions and it would seem that information, given in an appropriate way, may reduce the levels of stress experienced by young patients and that this, in turn, may have therapeutic benefits. (Some research suggests that the fact that stress levels are reduced may have an actual physical effect on the patient's immune and nervous systems.)

Meaning of participation

As to what is meant by 'participation', a variety of definitions exist reflecting both broad and narrow objectives. In the former sense, its link with democracy and citizenship is stressed (Hart, 1992), while in the latter, it is the input to individual decisions which is important (Save the Children, 2005). It is securing this opportunity for children to express their views and influence decision-making that is most closely reflected in Article 12 of the UNCRC. It is the implementation of this right in the healthcare setting which this research sets out to measure.

Although participation in the broadest sense involves a range of activities and circumstances, key factors to understanding the concept, according to Sinclair (2004), are:
- the level of engagement;
- the focus of the decisions;
- the nature of the activity;
- the children involved.

The *level of engagement* is a complex issue which is often described in terms of power-sharing between adults and children. Hart (1992) describes participation as stages on the rung of a ladder, where each step is associated with the degree to which children are in control of the process. According to Hart's Ladder of Participation, the bottom 3 rungs of the ladder — manipulation, decoration and tokenism — relate to non-participation, whereas rungs 4-8 involve increasing degrees of participation of children in decision-making processes — assigned but informed; consulted and informed; adult-initiated shared decisions with children; child-initiated and directed; and child-initiated shared decisions with adults.

While Hart's hierarchical model has been criticised for focusing on the need to strive for the top of the ladder regardless of the circumstances (Treseder, 1997), others have argued that different levels may be appropriate for different tasks as part of an activity or project (Shier, 2001). Treseder has adapted Hart's model of participation by categorising the degrees of participation (rungs 4-8) as different yet equal forms of good practice, so that the most appropriate form or level of participation may be chosen to suit each individual child's environment (Treseder, 1997). Shier has also developed a typology for child participation which relates specifically to the implementation of Article 12 of the UNCRC. According to Shier's model, the five levels of child participation are where children are listened to; children are supported in expressing their views; children's views are taken into account; children are involved in decision-making processes; and children share power and responsibility for decision-making (Shier, 2001).

While Shier envisages that all levels of participation are genuine, he maintains that Article 12 requires the participation of children at level three (where children's views are taken into account). He also usefully identifies three levels of commitment on the part of adults seeking to ensure the participation of children. The first degree of commitment — the opening — occurs once the adult is ready to take the views of the child into account. The second degree — the opportunity — arises when a decision-making process exists enabling the views of the child to be taken into account. The third and final degree of commitment — the obligation — is established when a policy decision is made to implement Article 12 and to effectively ensure that children's views are given due weight in decision-making.

With regard to the *focus of decisions* that affect children, a distinction is often made between private and public decisions. While public decisions include those relating to policy, public service provision and delivery, private decisions are often described as those made within the family environment and between individuals. However, they also include those made in private settings, including the healthcare environment *(see below)*.

The *nature of participation activity* can take many forms and includes one-off consultation exercises, ongoing involvement in the governance of institutions such as schools and participation in individual decision-making.

As regards the fourth key factor — *the children involved* — the UNCRC defines a child as everyone below the age of 18 years. Thus, participation of children under Article 12, by definition, includes children of all ages. This is supported further by an increased understanding of the capacity and competence of children to form and express views on matters relating to them. However, as Sinclair (2004) points out, it also emphasises the need to design approaches and forms of dialogue that facilitate engagement with children by starting with the position of the child, whatever their age or ability. As Sinclair highlights, what is crucial is that adults have an understanding of the complexities involved so that they can match the activity to its purpose; only then, she says, will they be in a position to engage honestly with children.

Participation of children in the public arena

To date, participation activity has focused primarily on involving children and young people in public decision-making and in both once-off and ongoing initiatives in areas of governance and policy development. For example, children's parliaments and youth advisory panels are commonplace in many countries (Lansdown, 2001), as is the involvement of children in the drafting of relevant policy documents on healthcare, welfare and education, and the making of strategic appointments.

In Ireland, young people were involved in the drafting of the National Children's Strategy in 2000 (NCO, 2000), in the appointment of the Ombudsman for Children in 2003 and in the development of a national set of child well-being indicators in 2005 (Hanafin and Brooks, 2005). However, in 2001 research indicated a low level of participation of young people more generally in the statutory sector, with their involvement being limited to consultation where their views were sought in adult-led groups (NYCI, 2001). The voluntary sector, in contrast, was found to engage with young people in a wide variety of ways, although the lack of resources explained the failure to document, fully integrate and evaluate the effectiveness of this work. Cultural barriers, particularly the perception that children and young people did not have the capacity to participate fully in decision-making, were also a clear factor *(ibid)*.

Toolkits and practice guides have been developed to help voluntary and statutory organisations involve young people in their work in a meaningful way (NCO *et al,* 2005; Lansdown, 2001). Best practice on genuine participation and 'good consultation' in the public area is now well documented and attention is beginning to shift to the mainstreaming of such best practice across the statutory and voluntary sector (McAuley and Brattman, 2002).

Participation of children in the private arena

By contrast, relatively little attention has focused on children's participation in the private arena. In children's rights terms, this may be explained by the now obsolete notion that private relations were excluded from the protection afforded by human rights law, which was originally considered to concern vertical relations between the State and its citizens, rather than horizontal relations between private individuals. This perception, combined with the veil of privacy that protects the family from outside interference, may explain the focus on the child's right to be heard in the public sector.

However, recognition of the enormous influence that the family has on children's lives and the clear acknowledgement that the child's rights are not suspended within the family environment have helped to shift attention on to the protection of children's rights in the private sphere. This is supported by the fact that Article 12 of the UNCRC makes no distinction between private or public decisions regarding the child's right to be heard and taken into account, requiring only that children be involved in 'all matters affecting the child' (Lansdown, 2001). The advantages as well as the barriers to the participation of children in decision-making can be measured equally on the private as well as the public side of the divide. Moreover, research shows both that children themselves value respect for their rights within the family and that involvement in family decision-making is a priority for them (Kilkelly *et al,* 2005).

Healthcare setting: A particular challenge
Decisions concerning children in the healthcare setting can have a significant impact on them (Phillips and Grahn-Farley, 2002). Such decisions are clearly ones that 'affect them' within the meaning of Article 12 of the UNCRC and thus the duty to listen to children and to take their views into account applies equally in this context.

Yet, research in the medical field suggests that children are not generally involved in their healthcare decisions. One study, for example, found that children are largely excluded from the interactions between parents and healthcare providers, and are generally not involved in discussions or decisions about their care (Angst and Deatrick, 1996). Another large US study found that children were seen as 'objects' that had things done to them rather than being involved in their treatment or having a voice (Knafl *et al,* 1998).

While this is perhaps ironic given that communication is such an essential feature of healthcare and one of the main roles of health professionals, it also highlights that implementing Article 12 in this setting is a particularly unique challenge. While a number of factors may explain why this is so, the complexity of the private, interpersonal relationship between health professional and patient, the child's perceived lack of capacity and the fact that a third party, such as a parent, may be involved when the patient is a child — all these can be seen to complicate the process of ensuring the child's voice is heard in the healthcare setting (McNeish and Newman, 2002).

Nature of the healthcare setting

The nature and history of the healthcare process raises particular difficulties in giving recognition to children's views. For example, it is only relatively recently that the views of capable, adult patients have begun to be taken into account. Historically, the physician's duty was to care for patients, to determine the most appropriate treatment for them and to dispense that treatment. The patient's views were considered an irrelevant part of the process. The prevailing ethic was a paternalistic one, essentially 'doctor knows best'.

Although patients now play a much greater role in their healthcare decisions, and consumerism has made its way into the healthcare setting to some extent, the residue of paternalism remains a feature of many aspects of healthcare. Some health professionals still find it difficult to recognise the essential role of patients in their own healthcare decisions. Some patients, too, prefer to leave the decision-making to their doctors and may be reluctant to engage with the process. Patients, especially those in hospital or with serious illness, may feel weak or vulnerable and may be disconcerted on finding themselves outside of their normal environment. For patients in this situation, participating in their healthcare decisions can be difficult, especially if the health professionals do not give the impression that they would welcome patient interaction.

Issues of capacity and consent and the role of health professionals

Vulnerability of the patient is exaggerated when the patient is a child of any age. Research shows that children are not typically involved in decisions made about their healthcare either legally or in practice (Phillips and Grahn-Farley, 2002). Moreover, doctors have traditionally seen child patients as 'incapable' of making healthcare decisions and this viewpoint has often been endorsed by parents giving doctors 'carte blanche to exclude their children from the decision-making process' (Gabe *et al*, 2004).

Yet, the view that child patients are 'incapable' suggests that, at some stage, they acquire the necessary capacity to participate in the consultation process. The problematic issue here is that the child's capacity is determined frequently by the health professionals who may have their own views, attitudes and perspectives on the child's capacity for partnership in this context. Moreover, there are no formal guidelines as to how health professionals should 'weigh up the interests of the child, the wishes of parents and the medical opinion of doctors' (Law Reform Committee, 2006). In addition, health professionals may not appreciate the importance of their own role in assisting the child, through effective communication and provision of age-appropriate information, to acquire the necessary level of capacity. The importance of training health professionals to communicate effectively with child patients, as well as raising awareness in the profession about the importance and value of the child's right to be heard, is patently clear in this context.

Role of parents and parental rights

The particular features of the patient-doctor relationship highlighted above are further complicated by a child's apparent or real immaturity and lack of legal capacity, which mean that the involvement of a third party (the parent or guardian) in the process is nearly always required. The extent of parental involvement and whether it is direct or indirect are important variables here and can distinguish between an essentially paternalistic approach to the child's healthcare — where the adults decide what is best for the child — and a rights-based approach — where the child is listened to and supported to be involved in the process. Moving from the former to the latter requires an acknowledgement that there are complex reasons for the differing views and attitudes of parents and professionals in this area which relate to perceptions of the parental right and need to protect their children, their awareness of the child's rights, the nature of their relationship with their children and what they may perceive as their unique understanding of the child's development, personality and health.

The impact of this complex dynamic on the treatment of children in the healthcare setting is well documented, as is the fact that health professionals and parents may be working towards different objectives. For example, Tates *et al* (2002) found that by taking into account the child's age, GPs are obviously striving for active child participation in medical communication. Parents, on the other hand, would appear to restrict child participation by interfering in doctor-child interactions, irrespective of the child's age.

Parents' tendency to obstruct rather than facilitate the participation of their children has also been recorded in other studies. According to Gabe *et al* (2004), 'sociological research in the 1970s and 1980s revealed that parents and doctors tended to discuss the child's illness without seeking to include the child's own point of view'. While some parents may now be more willing to encourage their children to participate in consultations around their healthcare, they often still act in an executive-like capacity, managing what and how their children are told about their illness (Young *et al,* 2003). Moreover, in the context of relations between GPs and child patients, Tates *et al* (2002) concluded that 'the low degree of child participation in the doctor-parent-child triad should not be interpreted as a sign of incompetence on behalf of the children, but rather as a consequence of the participants' underlying participation framework. We have to conclude that the adult participants play a pivotal role in enhancing or restricting child participation'.

This illustrates the power imbalance that militates against the child's right to participate being vindicated in the healthcare setting, where their subordination to parental authority is compounded by a feeling of inferiority to the health professional. The legal duty to vindicate the child's right to be heard is aimed at addressing this imbalance in favour of the child's participation in the process. For parents, however, this is not without difficulty, particularly when they may believe that giving rights to their children is a zero-sum game which sees them relinquish all parental power.

The rights of parents are given express recognition in Article 18 of the UNCRC, which also articulates the State's duty to provide appropriate assistance to parents in the exercise of parental responsibility. The principle of evolving capacity, set out in Article 5, is also relevant here insofar as it recognises the duty, right and responsibility of parents to guide their children in the exercise of their rights. According to this principle, parents, who exercise their rights on behalf of their young children, are encouraged to gradually cede these rights to their children as the child's willingness, capacity and development allows. This allows children to take on a more directly active and autonomous role in the decision-making process as they develop, although parents always retain ultimate responsibility for them and the decisions made. In this context, it is important to note that Article 12 does not provide for all children to have the final and decisive say, but that their views be given due weight in accordance with their age and maturity in preparation for adulthood, where their right to self-determination is complete.

Best practice: Involving children in their healthcare decisions

Despite the unique nature of the challenge to listen to children in the healthcare setting, little research has been undertaken into the implementation of Article 12 in this context. Few resources have been directed at the development of appropriate models and structures to ensure the voice of the child is heard in the healthcare setting. Moreover, the growth in children's participation activity in other areas has not been accompanied by the evaluation of the process of participation and thus very little analysis of the outcomes of participation from the child's perspective has been undertaken. To the extent that children's participation is a matter of right, Sinclair (2004) argues that it is 'not something that has to be justified by evidence or which needs to "prove" that it works'. However, research and analysis of consultation with children *is* important to ensure the most meaningful involvement of children in decisions made about their care and treatment.

While different models of participation will need to be developed for this setting, the same principles — of age-appropriate language and approaches, a genuine commitment to engage with young people and a willingness to take them seriously — must be shared by all adults in all settings if the child's rights are to be vindicated. Common too must be the objective to move from a child-focused approach to one that is child-centred: one which respects and values children; which treats each as an individual in his or her own right; which accords to them not only rights as children, but full human rights, equal with all others; and which sees every engagement with children as part of a jointly negotiated process (Sinclair, 2004).

While they may not have a rights-basis, a number of statements of best practice have been developed by health professionals with regard to the participation of children in the healthcare setting. In its *Good Medical Practice* guide, the Royal College of Paediatrics and Child Health requires paediatricians to respect the right of patients to be fully involved in decisions about their care (RCPCH, 2002). If the child is old enough to understand the nature, purpose and implications of their treatment, the paediatrician must, where possible, be satisfied that the patient has understood what is proposed and why, any significant risk associated with it, and have given consent. Failure to involve parents or carers or, where appropriate, the child is described as unacceptable practice (*ibid*, para. 17).

The RCPCH guide also sets out the requirements for good communication, which it describes as 'essential to effective care' (*ibid*, para. 21). Paediatricians are told that they must listen to children and young people and respect their views, and it is unacceptable practice to fail to listen appropriately to parents or carers or to override contrary views without adequate reason or explanation. Similarly, the Medical Council of Ireland in its *Guide to Ethical Conduct and Behaviour* (2004b) advises doctors that 'due regard must be had to the wishes of the child', but warns that the doctor must 'never assume that it is safe to ignore the parental/guardian interest'.

While clearly identifying the importance of communication, the guidance from the RCPCH and the Medical Council of Ireland does not give any real indication as to how good communication might be achieved. The final *Report of the Public Inquiry into Children's Heart Surgery at the Bristol Royal Infirmary 1984-1995*, published in 2001 by Bristol Royal Infirmary, addresses the matter of communication in more detail and its findings regarding best practice should be included in any statement of best practice in this area. The Bristol report notes that children, once they are no longer infants, are 'acute observers of the mood and body language of others ... It is impossible to avoid communicating with them'. Accordingly, it describes good practice as being founded on the principles of 'truthfulness, clarity and awareness of the child's age'. In practice, this means that health professionals who care for children must be able to listen to children, to respect their need for information and to be prepared to give information in the right amount and in a way that is suitable for the child's age. The report concedes that this is not always an easy or straightforward task and reiterates its conclusion — that all professionals dealing with children must be trained in paediatrics and in 'the special skill of communicating with children about illness and treatment'.

In developing its best practice on communication, the Bristol Royal Infirmary Inquiry (2001) drew heavily on a paper prepared for the Inquiry by Jean Simons, a Bereavement Services Co-ordinator at Great Ormond Street Hospital for Sick Children (Simons, 2000). Further practical insights into the operation of best practice may be gained from this work. Simons notes the importance of finding a suitable vocabulary, which does not involve 'talking down' to the child and yet which provides information in an age-appropriate way. She notes the usefulness of play specialists in communicating with very young children. She also notes difficulties with the use of euphemism around children based on the belief that this will be gentler or easier for the child to understand. Research suggests that euphemism (e.g. referring to 'going to heaven' rather than 'death') can be confusing and distressing for children.

Simons (2000) also notes research showing that the provision of information to children is not a once-off event. This research suggests that children's understanding changes with their physical, mental and psychological development and that information needs to be repeated, reiterated and discussed over a period of time. She also offers helpful advice on assessing children's information needs: she advises that the most effective way of assessing needs is to listen to the child and be guided by the child's questions. She argues that children will ask what they want to know and that they should be answered truthfully and clearly.

Arising from the above discussion, best practice in this area may be summarised as follows:

- the child must be involved in treatment decisions as far as possible;
- the patient's parents or carers must be involved in treatment decisions;
- the views of children must be obtained and respected;
- the relationship between healthcare professional and child should be based on truthfulness, clarity and awareness of the child's age;
- children must be listened to and their questions responded to, clearly and truthfully;
- communication with children is not a once-off occurrence, but must be an ongoing process;
- training in communication skills with children is an essential component of appropriate professional training.

2 THE CHILD'S RIGHT TO BE HEARD

UNDER ARTICLE 12 OF THE UN CONVENTION ON THE RIGHTS OF THE CHILD

The child's right to be heard, as set out in Article 12 of the UN Convention on the Rights of the Child (UNCRC), is at the heart of this research. Building on the discussion of children's participation rights *(see Chapter 1)*, this chapter aims to provide the legal, rights-based framework for the research by setting out the general meaning and scope of Article 12 and identifying the challenges involved in its implementation in the context of children's healthcare.

The following discussion of the legal basis for the requirement to listen to children is complemented by the guidance of the UN Committee on the Rights of the Child (the body responsible for monitoring implementation of the UNCRC), as well as by details of Ireland's progress in implementing Article 12.

Adopted by the United Nations in 1989, the UN Convention on the Rights of the Child is the most highly ratified human rights instrument in international law. It sets out the rights to which all children are entitled and represents strong international consensus on the treatment of children in all areas of their lives.

According to Hammarberg (1990), the UNCRC's provisions are often categorised under the headings of Protection, Provision and Participation. (Hammarberg also includes a fourth P for Prevention rights.)

- 'Protection' provisions include those rights that address the child's right to protection from harm and abuse. While the most important provision in this category is Article 19, which requires the State to take all measures to protect children from harm, abuse and ill-treatment, several other provisions (notably Articles 32-36) set out the right of the child to protection in other areas.
- The 'Provision' category of rights details the rights of the child to have his or her needs met, including the right to health and healthcare (Article 24), the right to an adequate standard of living (Article 27) and the right to education (Articles 28 and 29). It also provides for the right to play and leisure (Article 31) and makes provision for the rights of children with disabilities (Article 23), for children deprived of their family environment (Article 20) and refugee children (Article 22).
- The final group of rights falls under the 'Participation' heading. Spearheaded by Article 12, which recognises the child's right to be heard in all matters affecting him or her, the group contains fundamental civil rights such as the child's right to freedom of expression (Article 13), freedom of religion (Article 14) and freedom of association (Article 15). Also included in this category is the child's right to access appropriate information (Article 17) and the State's duty to make children and adults aware of children's rights (Article 42). These latter provisions have particular relevance to the area of healthcare *(see below)*.

Scope and significance of Article 12

The UN Committee on the Rights of the Child (referred to hereafter as 'the Committee') is the body responsible for monitoring the implementation of the UNCRC. According to the Committee, the UNCRC has four guiding principles which must inform its implementation in all areas (UN Committee on the Rights of the Child, 1996/2005; 2003). These are:

- The right to life, survival and development (Article 6).
- The principle of non-discrimination (Article 2). This guarantees Convention rights to all children without distinction.
- The best interests of the child (Article 3). This requires that in all decisions taken concerning children, the child's best interests must be a primary consideration.
- The right to be heard (Article 12).

The significance of identifying the child's right to be heard as one of the UNCRC's guiding principles is that it enjoys an elevated status within the framework of the Convention and its implementation. The pertinent part of Article 12 requires that:

> *1. States Parties shall assure to the child who is capable of forming his or her own views the right to express those views freely in all matters affecting the child, the views of the child being given due weight in accordance with the age and maturity of the child.*

The provision thus requires States to take measures to facilitate the child's expression of his or her views in all matters affecting him or her, and to ensure that those views are given due weight in accordance with the child's age and maturity. The two requirements of Article 12(1) are thus to facilitate expression of children's views and to have their views taken into account in accordance with their age and maturity. Both elements are limited only by the child's capacity to form his or her views, as opposed to the expression itself, and there is thus no lower age limit on the exercise of Article 12 rights. Nor do the dual criteria of 'age and maturity' limit the child's right to express his or her views: they merely apply to the weight to be given to those views.

In line with the view that very young children are capable of understanding and voicing their opinion on many issues, therefore, Article 12 recognises that competence does not develop along rigid time-lines or developmental stages. According to the Committee:

Young children are acutely sensitive to their surroundings and very rapidly acquire understanding of the people, places and routines in their lives, along with awareness of their own unique identity. They make choices and communicate their feelings, ideas and wishes in numerous ways, long before they are able to communicate through the conventions of spoken or written language. (UN Committee on the Rights of the Child, 2005)

In this regard, the duty to facilitate the exercise of every child's right to be heard is key and the wide application and relevance to children of all ages of the right to be heard is reinforced by Articles 1, 2 and 13 of the UNCRC. Article 1 defines a child as every human being below the age of 18 years, while Article 2 guarantees the enjoyment of Convention rights to all children without discrimination. The view that neither the right to be heard, nor the corresponding duty to listen to children is not limited to those capable of verbal communication, is further supported by Article 13, which recognises the child's right to freedom of expression 'either orally, in writing or in print, in the form of art, or through any media of the child's choice'.

Overall, therefore, Article 12 imposes a duty on all adults to listen to all children. Full implementation of Article 12 thus requires the use of a range of approaches and methods including verbal and non-verbal communication, using play, art and drawing, and the use of dolls and other props to communicate effectively with children. As to the areas in which this engagement must take place between adults and children, it is clear from the terms of Article 12 — which recognises the child's right to express his or her views 'in all matters affecting the child' — that the provision is to be broadly applied. The wide application of the principle to any area of activity or decision-making (including within the family and in other private settings) that affects the child is reinforced by the Committee's identification of the provision as one of the UNCRC's general principles.

Article 12 is thus a pivotal provision, which acknowledges the respect to which children are entitled and reflects their increasing autonomy and evolving capacity. Its implementation requires a 'profound and radical reconsideration of the nature of adult/child relationships' (Lansdown, 2001). Beyond the strict legal duty, the breadth and scope of Article 12 mean that it is a highly influential provision, which has the potential to bring about greater respect for children in their own right. In this way, Article 12 personifies what the UNCRC as a whole is trying to achieve for children.

The Committee has highlighted the relevance of Article 12 to all areas of the child's life, including in early childhood and in the public and private spheres (UN Committee on the Rights of the Child, 2005). It has also stressed its indivisibility from other related Convention provisions. In order to ensure that Article 12 is fully respected, Article 42 requires the State to make 'the principles and provisions of the Convention widely known by appropriate and active means to adults and children'. This duty to provide all children and adults with an awareness and an understanding of children's rights clearly extends to the child's right to be heard and requires that meaningful and age-appropriate public information campaigns be undertaken on a regular basis.

This is supported further by the duty in Article 4 to take all appropriate measures to implement the Convention and it is in this context that the Committee has consistently stressed the need for professional education and training to support the exercise by children of their rights (UN Committee on the Rights of the Child, 2003). In respect of young children, it has recommended that States take 'all appropriate measures to promote the active involvement of parents, professionals and responsible authorities in the creation of opportunities for young children to progressively exercise their rights within their everyday activities in all relevant settings, including by providing training in the necessary skills' (UN Committee on the Rights of the Child, 2005).

While children's right to know about their rights is given express protection in Article 42, recognition of the child's right to appropriate information under Article 17 is also crucial to the successful implementation of Article 12. While this provision refers chiefly to the responsibility of the mass media to disseminate information to children, it expressly guarantees the child's right to information from a diversity of sources, including those aimed at the promotion of the child's well-being and physical and mental health, making clear its relevance to the healthcare setting.

The final key provision here is Article 5, which enshrines the principles of parental guidance and evolving capacity. In particular, Article 5 requires the State to respect the responsibilities, rights and duties of parents to provide appropriate guidance and direction to the child in the exercise of his or her rights under the UNCRC. This makes it clear that while parents have a role to guide children in the exercise of their rights, this process must be undertaken in a manner consistent with the evolving capacity of the child (McGoldrick, 1991).

Implementation of Article 12

As outlined in Chapter 1, there are many advantages, including social, political and apparent medical or therapeutic reasons, for working towards a partnership model with children. It is, however, important to reiterate the legal nature of the duty to give the views of children due weight. The overriding requirement to implement the UNCRC can be found in Article 4, which requires States to take all appropriate legislative, administrative and other measures for its implementation.

The Committee set out in 2003 what States must do to secure effective implementation of the Convention in its *General Comment No. 5* (UN Committee on the Rights of the Child, 2003). Here, it noted that the development of a children's rights perspective throughout Government, Parliament and the judiciary is required for effective implementation of the whole Convention, but particularly for the general principles including Article 12. It also made a number of recommendations in the General Comment specific to the implementation of Article 12 in particular, highlighting the need to enshrine the principle in domestic law, to develop a national strategy to implement and monitor implementation of the Convention and to ensure that all those working with and for children undergo systematic and ongoing training and capacity building on the rights of children.

According to the Committee, it expects to see the Convention reflected in professional training curricula, codes of conduct and educational curricula at all levels (*ibid*, para. 53). Periodic evaluation of the effectiveness of children's rights training must also be undertaken, reviewing the knowledge of the Convention as well as the extent to which it has contributed to developing attitudes and practices that actively promote children's enjoyment of their rights. Incorporation of children's rights into the school curriculum is also vital in generating an awareness about children's rights among children themselves.

Further evidence as to the measures that must be taken to demonstrate effective implementation of Article 12 can be found in the Committee's *General Guidelines regarding the Form and Content of Periodic Reports* (1996/2005). These guidelines require States to submit information every 5 years on how Article 12 has been incorporated into legislation and how the views of children are incorporated into policy-making processes. They also require information on the measures taken to raise the awareness of families and the public in general on the need to encourage children to exercise their right to express their views and to train professionals working with children to encourage children to do so, and to give their views due weight.

The Committee's guidelines also contain specific requirements regarding the inclusion of the Convention, children's rights and child development issues in medical and nursing schools and in the broader curricula of health professionals. This serves to emphasise the relevance of children's rights, including their right to be heard, to the training and education of health professionals as a specific requirement of the legal duty to implement the UNCRC.

Other research in the area of children's rights has identified that health professionals need specialised training in obtaining the consent of children to all medical procedures, however minor, and in communicating effectively with and preparing children for any interventions made (Kilkelly *et al*, 2004). What is vital, however, is that these recommendations flow from a binding international duty to implement the UNCRC in good faith.

Ireland's implementation of Article 12

Ireland ratified the UNCRC without reservation on 28 September 1992 and it came into force one month later. Ireland is thus committed under international law to implementing the Convention's principles and provisions, including Article 12. However, since the UNCRC has not been incorporated into the domestic legal system in accordance with Article 29.6 of the Irish Constitution, it is not binding on agencies or bodies within the State. The UNCRC is thus binding on the State, but *not within it,* although limited statutory expression has been given to the duty to listen to the views of children and give them due weight in certain circumstances.

In particular, the duty is set out in the Child Care Act, 1991 and the Children Act, 2001, which make provision for the child to be heard in child care and criminal proceedings, respectively. The relevant sections of the Children Act, 1997, which amends the Guardianship of Infants Act, 1964 to provide for children to be separately represented in private family law proceedings, were never commenced. In addition, insofar as these laws provide for the child's right to be heard in judicial and administrative proceedings, they serve to implement the second, rather than the first paragraph of Article 12. The more general right of the child to have his or her views taken into account in all matters affecting him or her is completely absent from the statute books. Nor does this principle enjoy express Constitutional protection.

According to the Committee, the principle set out in Article 12 highlights the role of the child as an active participant in the promotion, protection and monitoring of his or her rights and it applies equally to all measures adopted by States to implement the Convention (UN Committee on the Rights of the Child, 2003). In 1998, following its consideration of Ireland's First Report on implementation of the UNCRC, the Committee expressed concern that Ireland's welfare policies and practices did not adequately reflect the child rights-based approach enshrined in the UNCRC (UN Committee on the Rights of the Child, 1998). It also expressed the view that insufficient steps had been taken to promote widespread awareness of the UNCRC and was concerned at the lack of adequate and systematic training on the principles and provisions of the UNCRC for professional groups, including health professionals, working with and for children (*ibid*, para. 11). Regarding the implementation of Article 12, the Committee expressed concern that the views of the child were not generally taken into account, including within the family, at schools and in society, and that procedures for hearing children were not fully considered in the legislation. In this regard, it recommended that the Irish Government take further measures to fully implement and incorporate Article 12 into domestic law and recommended that measures be taken to promote and facilitate children's participation and respect for their views in decisions and policies affecting them (*ibid*, para. 35).

Ireland submitted its Second Report to the Committee in July 2005 (Department of Health and Children, 2005). It will be examined in September 2006, when the Government will undoubtedly be commended for taking the following steps to implement the UNCRC: the adoption of the National Children's Strategy, the appointment of the Ombudsman for Children and the establishment of the Office of the Minister for Children.

National Children's Strategy

Subsequent to the Committee's 1998 criticism of Ireland's efforts to implement the UNCRC in general, and Article 12 in particular, the *National Children's Strategy: Our Children — Their Lives* was published in 2000 (Department of Health and Children, 2000). The Strategy was drafted following a public consultation process involving children and young people, as well as those working with and for them (NCO, 2000). The Strategy identified three national goals as follows:

- **Goal 1:** Children will have a voice in matters which affect them and their views will be given due weight in accordance with their age and maturity.
- **Goal 2:** Children's lives will be better understood; their lives will benefit from evaluation, research and information on their needs, rights and the effectiveness of service.
- **Goal 3:** Children will receive quality supports and services to promote all aspects of their development.

In addition to the commitment to listening to children shown by its drafters, the National Children's Strategy is also to be commended for singling out implementation of Article 12 as a national priority (Goal 1). While clearly, according to the Committee on the Rights of the Child, Ireland had much to do to implement fully the spirit and letter of Article 12 of the UNCRC (and the potential of the National Children's Strategy has yet to be measured in this respect), it is important nonetheless that the Strategy identifies giving children a voice as a national policy goal. More recently, this has influenced the National Play Policy, the objectives of which include giving children a voice in the design and implementation of play policies and facilities, a duty which is imposed on local authorities as well as on the National Children's Office (NCO, 2004).

It is also important that the National Children's Strategy makes a commitment to an evidence- and research-based approach to the development of law and policy on children's rights and services (Goal 2). This commitment forms the basis for the NCO's research programme, under which this project has been funded, and is to be widely welcomed.

Ombudsman for Children

The establishment of the Office of Ombudsman for Children, under the Ombudsman for Children Act 2002, represents another important milestone in the implementation of the State's duty to listen to children under Article 12 of the UNCRC. The Office has the important function of promoting the rights and welfare of children and also enjoys significant powers of examination and investigation of complaints and child-proofing of legislation, policy and practice (Martin, 2004). While exclusions from the complaints remit of the Office (e.g. children in certain places of detention) are worrisome, for the purposes of this research it is important that children in the healthcare system clearly fall within the Ombudsman's remit. Moreover, the credentials of the present incumbent, Emily Logan, who is an experienced children's nurse, mean that she is particularly well placed to maximise the potential of the Ombudsman's function to promote the rights of children in the healthcare setting.

Office of the Minister for Children

In addition to developments in these two significant areas, the recently established Office of the Minister for Children (OMC), of which the National Children's Office (NCO) is now part, has made a commitment to leading on children and young people's participation within the context of the National Children's Strategy. Heretofore, the NCO had established the Children and Young People's Forum to advise it on its work under the Strategy and published national guidelines in 2005, entitled *Young Voices: Guidelines on how to involve children and young people in your work* (NCO *et al*, 2005).

Summary

This chapter set the primary legal context for the right of children to be heard in the healthcare setting by explaining briefly the scope and purpose of Article 12 of the UN Convention on the Rights of the Child and highlighting the legal duty to implement the principle. It also introduced the concepts that underpin many of the primary research findings set out in the following chapters — the child's right to be heard, the duties of parental guidance and evolving capacity. Placing the duty to listen to children in the context of Ireland's international human rights obligations is vital, as is the need to reflect on its implementation within the framework of Irish law and policy.

3 CHILDREN, CONSENT AND THE LAW IN IRELAND

While Chapter 2 considered the children's rights framework for children's participation in healthcare decision-making, this chapter looks at the broader legal framework surrounding healthcare decisions and, in particular, the role of legal consent as it applies to children. It sets out the legal rules regarding consent and the obligations that the law places on health professionals, explaining the background to these rules and how they impact on the subject of this research.

The discussion begins by looking in brief at the role of consent in law. It then examines the question of whose consent is required when the patient is a child, looking at the legal role of parents and the legal rights of the child who is unable to give consent on his or her own behalf. The discussion ends with an examination of the factors that make consent meaningful, in particular, the role of information and the importance of communication between health professionals, patients and parents.

The issue of acquiring formal consent to medical intervention is necessarily a technical and legal one. In the context of children, the process of seeking and giving consent is undertaken principally between the child's parent and the health professional. As this research illustrates, however, obtaining the consent of the child to any medical procedure or intervention is considered by many health professionals to represent best practice. It is certainly at the heart of respect for the autonomy of children and for their right to bodily integrity. It is also essential to the relationship of trust that must exist between any health professional and their patient, although the vulnerability of children means that it has heightened relevance and importance in this context. While the issue of legal or formal consent is the focus of this chapter, therefore, the issues raised are also relevant to the more general issue of consent to intervention *(for detailed discussion, see Chapter 7)*.

Role of consent in law

The requirement to obtain consent to medical interventions is recognised by the law as being of fundamental importance. The requirement for legal consent comes from the law's recognition of the individual's right to autonomy or self-determination. In the words of a leading American judge: 'Every human being of adult years and sound mind has a right to determine what shall be done with his own body.' [1]

For the last two decades in particular, the law has accorded central importance to the right to autonomy and with this, it has been recognised that health professionals must obtain patient consent for any form of medical treatment (Donnelly, 2002). This means that (outside of certain limited circumstances, such as emergency surgery) medical intervention without legal consent will be held to constitute an unlawful interference with the patient's body and the health professional may be held responsible in the law of tort.

Traditionally, medical intervention without legal consent gave rise to an action in the tort of battery. Battery is a strict liability tort in that there is no need for a claimant to show that the health professional deliberately failed to obtain legal consent or even that he or she was negligent. The mere fact that legal consent was not given to the procedure is enough. The further important feature of battery is that there is no need to establish harm to a patient. Thus, even if a patient's condition is improved by the procedure, the health professional can still be liable in the tort of battery simply because of an absence of consent.

As will be seen below, the legal action of a failure to obtain consent to a procedure has now shifted away from the tort of battery and is instead located within the tort of negligence. This has the practical effect of making it more difficult for patients to pursue a legal action against health professionals because the action in negligence requires that the patient has suffered harm and that this harm is caused by the absence of proper consent.

Much of the legal protection of the right to autonomy presumes that the patient is an adult with full mental capabilities. Where the patient is a young child or has significant intellectual

---

[1] *Schloendorff v Society of New York Hospital* (1914) 211 NY 125, 128.

disabilities, the right to autonomy applies in a different way and, in particular, the patient's freedom to decide what should be done with his or her body is not accorded the same status. With children, the requirement for consent still remains important. However, usually somebody acting on behalf of the child gives legal consent and not the child himself. For children, most of the time, this person will be the child's parent.

Whose legal right to consent?

The first issue to clarify in relation to legal consent in the case of children is whose consent is required. At what point does a child or young person attain the legal right to consent to treatment? A further question on this point is whether the fact that a young person has the legal right to consent will automatically mean that he or she also has the legal right to refuse treatment.

Section 23 of the Non-Fatal Offences against the Person Act, 1997 states that a person aged more than 16 years may give consent to 'surgical, medical or dental' treatment. The Section continues by providing that 'where a minor has by virtue of this section given an effective consent to any treatment it shall not be necessary to obtain any consent for it from his or her parent or guardian'. 'Surgical, medical or dental treatment' is defined in Section 23(2) as including 'any procedure undertaken for the purposes of diagnosis'. The Section also applies to 'any procedure (including in particular the administration of an anaesthetic) which is ancillary to any treatment as it applies to that treatment'.

Section 23 does not set out the position regarding children aged less than 16 years nor does it explicitly state that children aged more than 16 years may refuse treatment. It is therefore necessary to look outside the Act to attempt to determine the answers to these questions.

The legal position of children under the age of 16 is unclear. In the UK, in the case of *Gillick v West Norfolk and Wisbech AHA*[2], the House of Lords held that a child aged less than 16 (the statutory age for consent in the UK) could legally consent to medical treatment provided the child had 'sufficient maturity' to make the decision in question. The treatment at issue in *Gillick* itself was contraceptive treatment. (Mrs. Gillick had asked her local health authority to give an undertaking that they would not prescribe the contraceptive pill to any of her five daughters without her prior consent.)

The importance of *Gillick* lies in the fact that it removed an age or 'status'-based limit regarding who can consent to treatment and introduced instead an individualised test whereby each child's capacity to consent is tested, usually by a doctor or other member of the medical profession. *Gillick* was commonly regarded as a significant step forward in recognising adolescent autonomy and according a voice to some children in relation to their healthcare decisions. Some commentators have noted, however, that *Gillick* in fact handed over power from parents to the medical profession, in that the young person's right to consent was dependent on a member of the medical profession determining that the young person in question was capable.

Two important limits on the effect of *Gillick* should be noted. First, the standard of maturity laid down by the courts is a high one. Lord Scarman set out the standard for maturity (in the particular circumstances of contraceptive treatment) as follows: 'There is much that has to be understood by a girl under the age of 16 if she is to have legal capacity to consent to such treatment. It is not enough that she should understand the nature of the advice which is being given: she must also have a sufficient maturity to understand what is involved. There are moral and family questions, especially her relationship with her parents; long-term problems associated with the emotional impact of pregnancy and its termination; and there are the risks to health of sexual intercourse at her age, risks which contraception may diminish but cannot eliminate.'[3]

---

[2] [1986] AC 112.

[3] *ibid*, p. 189.

Secondly, in two later decisions, the Court of Appeal held that while children under the age of 16 can give consent to treatment, children and young people up to the age of 18 cannot refuse their consent to treatment.[4] Thus, if a child or young person under the age of 18 refuses treatment, their parent or guardian may override their wishes and give a legally binding consent on their behalf. If the parent declines to do this, the court has ultimate authority to give consent on behalf of the child if it considers that the treatment in question is in the child's best interests.

The Irish courts have not yet considered any of these questions and the position here is complicated by the Constitution of Ireland. Article 41 of the Constitution gives rights to the family (based on marriage) and Article 42 states that parents have an inalienable right and duty to provide for the 'religious and moral, intellectual, physical and social education of their children'. These parental rights and duties could be held to limit a young person's freedom to consent to treatment such as contraception which, it might be argued, has an impact on the religious, moral and social education of children.

As against this, a young person also has rights under the Constitution of Ireland, including a right to privacy under Article 40.3.1. Even if a court were to limit the right of a young person to consent to contraceptive treatment, it is probable that a court would hold that a young person under the age of 16 can consent to other forms of treatment provided that the young person is shown to have the necessary maturity.

In relation to a young person's refusal of treatment, it is more difficult to predict what an Irish court would do. On the one hand, it might be argued that according a young person a right to consent to treatment is meaningful only if he or she also has the right to refuse. However, a court might also conclude that treatment refusal raises particular difficulties, especially if the refusal puts a young person's life in danger.

The children considered in this research are aged approximately between 6 and 12 years. This means that, in most cases, they are unlikely to be found to be sufficiently mature to give legal consent. The English cases following *Gillick* have tended to concern children aged 14 years or more. From a legal point of view, therefore, it is most likely that legal consent will be obtained from the child or young person's parent(s) or guardians. This does not mean, of course, that the child has no legal rights or indeed that the issue of whether the child consents does not still arise (*see below*). Nor does it mean that a child within the age group considered by this research could never be found to have the right to give a personal consent. The whole essence of an individualised test to decide if a child is sufficiently mature to give consent is that decisions are made about each young person rather than simply on the basis of age. For the majority of children and young people covered by this research, however, it is necessary to look next at the legal role of the parent(s) or guardians.

Consent: The role of parents

In general, under Irish law parents can consent to treatment and refuse treatment on behalf of their child. However, this right is limited to a degree. In the case of *North Western Health Board v HW and CW* [5], the Supreme Court set out some of the limits on parents' rights. The parents in this case refused to give their consent to the PKU test (commonly known as the 'heel' test) being carried out on their child because they did not agree with puncturing the child's blood vessel.

The Supreme Court held that the parents had the right to refuse the procedure. The parents' rights were protected by Article 42 of the Constitution. This Article recognises the family as the 'primary and natural educator of the child' and goes on to state that the State may supply the place of the parents only in 'exceptional circumstances' where the parents 'for physical or moral reasons fail in their duty towards their children'.

---

[4] *Re R. (A Minor)* [1991] 4 All E.R. 177 and *Re W. (A Minor)* [1992] 4 All E.R. 627.

[5] [2001] 3 IR 622.

In this case, the parents' refusal to consent to the procedure did not come within the category of exceptional circumstances. Therefore, the refusal did not justify the State (or the medical profession) in interfering with the parents' rights. In the words of Justice Denham: 'Every day, all over the State, parents make decisions relating to the welfare, including physical, of their children. Having received information and advice they make a decision. It may not be the decision advised by the doctor (or teacher, or social worker, or psychologist, or priest, or other expert) but it is the decision made, usually responsibly, by parents and is abided by as being in the child's best interests.' [6]

The Supreme Court set out a test to determine when a parents' right to make decisions for their child would be limited. Justice Denham described the test as follows: 'The test involves the weighing of all the circumstances, including parental responsibility, parental decisions, the child's personal rights, and the rights of all persons involved with and in the family, to determine in these circumstances what is in the best interests of the child.' [7] In the circumstances, the refusal of the PKU test did not place the child at risk to an extent sufficient to merit interference with the parents' rights.

In a later case, the High Court held that refusal of a blood transfusion by parents who were Jehovah's Witnesses did constitute 'exceptional circumstances' and permitted the hospital to provide the treatment to the child even though the parents refused.[8]

Parents' right to make decisions on behalf of their child is also protected under the European Convention on Human Rights (ECHR), recently incorporated into Irish law by the ECHR Act 2003. In the case of *Glass v United Kingdom*[9], the European Court of Human Rights held that the United Kingdom was in breach of Article 8 of the ECHR (which protects the right to private life) arising from a case involving a boy of 14 years who had severe intellectual and physical disabilities. The hospital in the case had placed a 'Do Not Resuscitate' (DNR) order on the boy's file without his mother's knowledge and contrary to the boy's family's expressed wishes. The hospital also administered the pain-relieving drug diomorphine to the boy contrary to his mother's wishes. The mother did not wish this drug to be administered because she feared that its use would speed up the boy's death.

The European Court of Human Rights found that the hospital's action in imposing treatment on the boy was in breach of his right to private life, in particular his right to physical integrity. This did not mean that the hospital could never take this kind of action; however, before a decision could be taken to impose or withdraw treatment contrary to the wishes of a parent, a facility should exist whereby the matter could be decided by a court and not solely by the medical profession.

The cases set out above are, by and large, exceptional. Most of the time, parents and medical professionals do not disagree regarding the appropriate treatment for the child. However, if there is a disagreement, the case law suggests that health professionals must obtain court approval before proceeding with procedures or treatment contrary to the wishes of the parents.

Consent: The role of the child

Even very young children may have strong views on whether or not they wish to have a procedure or treatment. Children's responses to proposed procedures may range from agreement through unenthusiastic assent, moderate disagreement to full-scale rejection. Children may have complex reasons for their responses; sometimes they may not be able to explain why they feel as they do. The challenges faced by children, parents and health professionals are discussed in detail in Chapters 5, 6 and 7, respectively.

---

[6] [2001] 3 IR 622, p.723.

[7] *ibid*, p. 725.

[8] See *The Irish Times,* 6 August 2004. The decision of Abbott J. was not reported and the parties were not publicly identified.

[9] [2004] ECHR 102.

The fact that a parent has the formal legal power to give consent for a child who is not legally capable does not mean that the child's consent is irrelevant. Nor does it mean that health professionals can simply force treatment on unwilling children. The fact that a child is incapable of consenting to treatment does not mean that the child's fundamental constitutional rights can be disregarded. In the case of *In re a Ward of Court*[10], the Supreme Court held that the individual rights of incapable patients (in this case, a woman in a persistent vegetative state) must be protected in the same way as the rights of capable patients. In *Re Article 26 and the Adoption (No. 2) Bill 1987*[11], the Supreme Court held that the rights of the child who is a member of a family are not limited to the family-based protections set out in Articles 41 and 42 of the Constitution of Ireland, but that the child also has personal rights under Article 40.3 of the Constitution.

Article 40.3.1 of the Constitution provides the basis for a range of unenumerated (or unstated) rights which are relevant in the context of healthcare and treatment. These rights include the right to dignity, the right to bodily integrity and the right to autonomy or self-determination. The Irish courts have not yet considered how these rights might impact on the medical treatment of children. However, there is a strong argument to be made that, even if a child cannot consent on his or her own behalf, certain kinds of behaviour towards the child may infringe these rights. For example, using physical means in order to force a reluctant child to comply with a medical procedure may, in some circumstances, constitute a breach of the child's right to bodily integrity, even if the child's parents have consented to the treatment. This does not mean that a child could never be forced to have a procedure. However, in such circumstances, it could be considered necessary to show that any imposition of treatment is in the best interests of the child and that there is no other, less invasive, means of providing the treatment in question. This is recognised by some professionals in practice *(see Chapter 7)*.

Informed consent: The role of information

The right to information

The relationship of information to participation was introduced earlier, in Chapter 2. Moreover, it is a fundamental legal principle that, in order to be meaningful, consent must be based on the provision of adequate information. This means that the patient must be given certain basic information relating to the procedure to which his or her consent is required, including information about the nature of the procedure and any risks involved. The term 'informed consent' is sometimes used to express this requirement.

The legal obligation to provide certain basic information remains in force even when the consent is given on behalf of another person, such as where a parent gives consent on behalf of a child. Failure to provide information may lead to the health professional being found liable in the tort of negligence and, provided that the claimant can show that he or she was harmed by the absence of the information (for example, that he or she would have acted differently if the information in question had been known), may lead to an award of damages in the claimant's favour.

What information?

In *Bolton v Blackrock Clinic*[12], the Supreme Court held that a patient is legally entitled to the information that a reasonable doctor would consider appropriate to give to a patient. In the later High Court case of *Geoghegan v Harris*[13], the court took a rather different approach. Here, the necessary information was described as the information that a reasonable patient would want to know. In most cases, there is very little difference between the two standards. A reasonable doctor will usually consider it appropriate to disclose information that a reasonable patient would want to know. Most Irish (and international) cases in this area have been concerned with the obligation to

---

[10] [1996] 2 IR 79.

[11] [1989] IR 656.

[12] Unreported Supreme Court, 23 January 1997.

[13] Unreported High Court, 21 June 2000.

give information about the risks in a treatment and specifically with the question of what level of risk must be brought to the patient's attention. The Irish courts have not yet considered in detail whether there is a legal obligation to provide information about such matters as alternative treatments and the relative benefits of treatments.

Whose right? The parent's right to information

When a parent is required to give consent to treatment on behalf of a child, it is reasonable to expect that the parent be given information of an equivalent level to that which they would receive if they were giving consent on their own behalf. In *Quinn v The South Eastern Health Board*[14], O'Caoimh J. held that a consent given by a 14-year-old girl to a neurological procedure was not an informed consent because neither the girl nor her parents had been advised on the risks associated with the procedure. These included the risks involved if the procedure failed and, in particular, the fact that such failure would reduce the possibility for other, more conservative treatment being followed.

The importance of providing adequate information to parents who are giving consent on behalf of their children was made clear in the Report issued by the Bristol Royal Infirmary Inquiry (2001). This public inquiry was concerned with a range of issues relating to the way in which paediatric heart surgery was carried out at the Bristol Royal Infirmary and was initiated because of an unusually high death rate among infant patients in the hospital.

The inquiry uncovered a number of problems in organisation, care and communication. According to the report, parents stated that communication between the cardiac team and parents was poor. Informing parents about the treatment and about their options seemed to be regarded as something of a chore. In particular, parents expressed unhappiness about the level of information provided to them about risks and alternatives. The inquiry also found that cardiologists had sometimes deliberately painted a falsely optimistic picture of a child's prognosis in order to keep up parents' hopes.

The Report of the Bristol Royal Infirmary Inquiry (2001) noted the importance of partnership between parents, patients and health professionals. Its Recommendation No. 15 confirmed that it was best practice that parents with a child in hospital should be involved in their child's care and that the involvement of the parents (as the people who know the child best and who care for the child) had to be 'fully acknowledged and appropriately engaged'.

Whose right? The child's right to information

Although a child may not be legally capable of giving consent to a procedure, he or she may still have a legal right to information. Unfortunately, the courts in Ireland have not yet considered this issue in detail. In *Quinn v The South Eastern Health Board* (discussed above), the Judge held that a 14-year-old girl's consent to a neurological procedure was not informed because neither the girl nor her parents were given adequate information. This seems to suggest that the girl herself had a personal entitlement to information. However, as the matter was not considered in more detail, the legal position remains unclear.

There are a number of reasons why a child should have a personal right to information relating to healthcare decisions. First, as noted above, the child's legal rights are not dependent on the child having legal capacity. It can be argued that it is overly simplistic to view the duty to disclose as being directed towards the person who has legal capacity to consent and not to include the actual patient within the ambit of the duty. As noted above, the courts recognise that children and young people mature at different rates and can be considered capable of different functions at different stages. Just because a young person is not sufficiently mature to consent to medical treatment does not mean that he or she cannot understand information relating to the treatment proposed, formulate a view on the treatment in question and have an entitlement to know the nature of the procedure proposed.

---

[14] Unreported High Court, 22 March 2002.

Chapters 5, 6 and 7 of this report explore these issues from the perspectives of children, parents and health professionals, respectively, and demonstrate that children who have had a lot of interaction with the healthcare professions, usually because of their medical conditions, are capable of formulating views and understanding proposed treatment from a young age.

Another reason why a child should have a personal right to information relating to healthcare decisions involves a therapeutic argument favouring the provision of information. There is a body of empirical research on informed consent that indicates that patients who have been involved with their healthcare decisions, including having more full information, tend to have a better response to treatment (Fallowfield *et al,* 1990). Although this work has for the most part been concerned with adults, children may also experience benefits from greater levels of involvement in their healthcare decisions. This view is supported by this research.

Making sense of information

The simple provision of information to a patient (or parent) does not ensure that the patient will understand or make sense of the information given. This is all the more true when a patient is a child or young person. The obligation to provide information must take account of the need to make information accessible to the patient. Otherwise, the consent of a patient (or parent) is nominal only. The courts in Ireland have not dealt in any detail with the issue of how accessible information should be. Instead, the main legal preoccupation has been with the amount of information to be given.

There are special challenges in making information accessible to children and young people. Those interviewed for this research provide a range of suggestions for ways in which health professionals should deal with the task of providing information *(see also Chapter 2)*. These issues, along with the issue of consent, are explored further in the following chapters.

Summary

This chapter examined the law relating to consent to healthcare treatment. As seen, consent is an essential legal requirement for treatment. For the many children who are unable to give personal consent, the consent of their parents should be obtained. However, the parental right to make treatment choices for their children is not absolute and parents' views regarding the most appropriate treatment may be overridden in 'exceptional circumstances'.

It has also argued that simply because a child is not legally capable of consenting to treatment does not mean that treatment may be imposed on the child. The child has rights protected under the Constitution — to autonomy, to bodily integrity and to dignity — and these rights are not dependent on the child having legal capacity to consent. On this basis, it was argued that the imposition of treatment on a resistant child is something which should be approached with great care and that matters such as the child's best interests and the least invasive alternative should be taken into account.

The final point made in this chapter related to the provision of information — the legal concept of 'informed consent'. It was argued that the legal entitlement to information is not necessarily restricted to adult patients, but that children also have an entitlement to information, even if they are not necessarily able to give legal consent to a procedure. The way in which all of these legal issues are dealt with in clinical practice will be discussed later.

4 METHODOLOGY

Objectives

The principal aim of the research was to explore the extent to which the voice of the child is heard in the Irish healthcare setting in line with Article 12 of the UN Convention on the Rights of the Child. Its objectives were:

- to consider the extent to which children are listened to by health professionals;
- to identify the obstacles to listening and communicating with children in the healthcare setting;
- to identify best practice in the area and to make proposals as to how it can be mainstreamed.

These objectives were pursued by the use of three main research approaches: a literature review and the collection of primary data to record a 'snapshot' of the experiences, views and attitudes of children, parents, and health professionals to the issue of child participation in the healthcare setting. In addition, a curriculum review was undertaken to establish a children's rights audit of the education and training curricula of health professionals. An overview of each research approach is given below, following by the ethical considerations involved.

The key strength of the research is thus the combination of a range of stakeholder perspectives, together with a curriculum audit, to advance a unique and focused understanding of the issue addressed.

For the purposes of this research, 'the healthcare setting' was broadly defined to include all environments or places in which children's healthcare is addressed in the community and in hospitals by medical practitioners, dentists, nurses and therapists.

Literature review

A review was undertaken of the literature on children's rights and medical law concerning the child's right to be heard in the healthcare setting and to have their views taken into account in accordance with their age and maturity. The issue of legal consent was also researched as a separate, but related issue.

The literature review established the framework of the research and identified the theoretical benchmarks against which the empirical findings could be measured. By focusing on the rights of the child in this area and the legal issue of consent, it also offered a legal context and background to the study. This framework is set out in Chapters 2 and 3.

Curriculum review

An evaluation was conducted of the education and training curricula of a number of health professions for compliance with the requirements of Article 12 of the UN Convention on the Rights of the Child and the extent to which they incorporated children's rights and communication with children.

The curriculum review was designed to identify whether the training of health professionals addressed the child's right to be heard and included best practice regarding how to communicate effectively with children. To this end, interviews with health professionals were supplemented by a review of educational curricula.

The curriculum review focused mainly on the undergraduate courses in medicine, nursing and dentistry, which are taught at the five principal medical schools — University College Cork, University College Dublin, National University of Ireland Galway (NUIG), Trinity College Dublin, and the Royal College of Surgeons. The review included a survey of relevant post-graduate courses, specialising in areas such as speech and language therapy and occupational therapy. It also attempted to research the clinical education, which completes the training of those entering the medical profession, provided under the aegis of the Medical Council of Ireland.

Some difficulties were encountered during this part of the research. First, while it was possible to identify the broad curriculum pursued at undergraduate level, it proved difficult to obtain the full details or content of the courses followed. Thus, while it was possible to identify that medical students at NUIG took a course in Communications or Ethics, for example, it was not always possible to determine the content of these courses and, in particular, whether they included the subject of communicating with children or parents. In this regard, course details were frequently noted to be 'unavailable' or course content described as 'under review'.

Secondly, the education and training of the medical profession is, to a large extent, provided through the process of clinical education or on-the-job training. Since this training is largely unstructured and does not always follow a set curriculum, it proved difficult to obtain written documentation on the subjects followed or to determine whether and how the skills of communicating and consulting with children were taught.

Interviews with health professionals compensated in some way for the lack of syllabus information. Accordingly, their views on education and training provided an important complement to this part of the research. Because of these limits, the research focuses primarily on the medical profession. More extensive research is thus required to produce a more comprehensive understanding of the education and training curricula of all health professionals in Ireland.

Collection of primary data

A number of individual and group interviews were held with children, parents and health professionals. NGOs and other support groups were also invited to make submissions to the research.

Rationale for the approach taken

The primary aim of this research was to record a snapshot of the extent to which children are listened to in the healthcare setting from the perspectives of children, parents and health professionals. Time and resource constraints required that careful consideration was given as to how best to record these perspectives. In all cases, the choice of research methods was determined by the fact that this was an exploratory study. Accordingly, the decision was made to focus on the collection of qualitative data and to undertake this part of the research by means of individual and group interviews. While other approaches, such as questionnaires, were considered, it was clear that a methodology which incorporated both individual and group interviews provided the best opportunity to gather rich and meaningful data from a relatively small number of participants (Hill *et al,* 1996). The interview model is flexible enough to be adapted to the circumstances and the needs of individual participants, and to use a variety of interview techniques, such as picture cards for young children.

The Sample

Given the exploratory nature of this research and the time constraints under which it was conducted, convenience sampling was used to identify participants. Children and parents were accessed through NGOs working with children and/or in the healthcare setting, and included children who had experienced standard or typical levels of contact with the healthcare setting, as well as those who had experienced higher levels of contact due to serious illness. Health professionals were also identified using the convenience method and the snowball technique was also used.

Although there are limitations to these methods (in particular, it is difficult to identify how representative the sample is), the inclusion of a range of ages and genders among the children, as well as some diversity in background and geographical location in all categories, reduces these limitations somewhat. Clearly, however, more extensive research is required to present a more detailed understanding of the issues addressed here.

Children and young people

As this research aimed to record a broad snapshot of children's experiences, rather than to represent the views of children in hospital or particularly sick children, the principal selection criterion used was age *(see Table 1)*. The range used was 5 to 14 years, and is well supported by the research literature (Angst and Deatrick, 1996; Sartain *et al,* 2000; King and Cross, 1989) and other factors, such as the age at which consent to medical treatment is relevant. In total, 51 children were interviewed, including children who had typical or average levels of experience of health professionals (the 'General' category listed in Table 1) and those who had more intense or long-term involvement with the healthcare system due to serious illness (the 'Serious illness' category in Table 1). A broad geographical representation was achieved, with children interviewed in Cork, Limerick, Dublin, Dundalk, Longford and Waterford, from urban and rural locations, and from different backgrounds.

Table 1: Number, ages, gender and health condition of children interviewed

Transcript No.	Category	Number and ages of children	Gender
1	General	2 children, aged 8 and 10	2 boys
2	General	6 children, aged 8-11	2 girls, 4 boys
3	General	4 children, aged 5-7	4 boys
4	General	6 children, aged 5, 6, 7, 9, 11 and 12	2 girls, 4 boys
5	General	7 children, aged 7, 8, 8, 9, 10, 10 and 11	2 girls, 5 boys
6	General	5 children, aged 8, 9, 9, 10 and 12	4 boys, 1 girl
7	Serious illness	1 child, aged 11	1 boy
8	Serious illness	1 child, aged 10	1 boy
9	Serious illness	1 child, aged 6	1 boy
10	Serious illness	3 children, aged 8, 8 and 11	3 boys
11	Serious illness	5 children, aged 6, 10, 12, 13 and 13	4 girls, 1 boy
12	Serious illness	6 children, aged 5, 8, 10, 11, 11 and 12	1 girl, 5 boys
13	General	3 children, aged 13, 14 and 14	3 girls
14	General	1 child, aged 12	1 girl

Parents

The research involved interviews with 30 parents of children between the ages of 5 and 14, and included parents whose children had not experienced any significant illness as well as those who had. The majority of parents (19) were related to the children interviewed. They were generally identified using the same approaches described above and achieved the same geographical representation. In addition, a group of parents from the Traveller community was included.

Health professionals

Convenience sampling was used to identify health professionals for participation in the research insofar as a list was drawn up identifying four categories, representation of which was considered essential for the purposes of the research. These were general practitioners (GPs, nurses and dentists); front-line staff of Accident and Emergency units (A&E professionals); consultants; and children specialists. Initial contact was made with a number of key health professionals in each category who agreed to be interviewed; they also identified colleagues where this was necessary to fill gaps in the sample.

In total, 22 health professionals were interviewed on an individual basis, including children's specialists and practitioners of general medicine (GPs), both in the hospital setting and in the community. The sample consisted of GPs (2); dentists (2); nurses (4); play specialists (2); psychologist (1); radiographer (1); A&E doctor (1); social workers (2); anaesthetists (3); dermatologists (2); and ENT consultants (2).

Three group interviews were also conducted with the (mainly nursing) staff of a children's unit and medical interns at two hospitals, and a range of health professionals involved in education and training at a medical school. This brought the total number of professionals interviewed to 50. The geographical spread covered Cork, Dublin and Sligo, and Counties Tipperary and Galway.

Interviews with children

In total, 14 interviews were carried out, consisting of individual (4) and group interviews (10). Vignettes, picture cards and story boards were all developed for children aged 5-8 and 9-11 respectively, since these were considered the most appropriate and efficient way to explore these issues with these age groups. They aimed to introduce different healthcare settings to the children, to explain the objectives of the research and to prompt discussion on the issues of communication and participation, and their experiences of these with health professionals.

Having obtained the consent of both children and parents prior to conducting the interviews, the interviews began by each child explaining the number of times they had been to the doctor, dentist or hospital. This enabled the research to take into account the experiences of those children:
- who were very sick or had long-term illness;
- who had low level but ongoing health problems;
- who had visited A&E units;
- who had visited their GP, health nurse or dentist.

In order to achieve the objectives of the research, the principal issues on which the children's views were sought were identified as follows:
- Do children like visiting their (a particular) dentist, doctor, the hospital, etc? What do/did they like or dislike about the visit? Was it frightening? Fun? Scary? If so/not why?
- Did the doctor/dentist/nurse talk to them, to the accompanying parent or both? How did this make them feel?
- Were the children able to understand everything the doctor/dentist/nurse said to their parent or to them? Did they ask any questions? Did they feel they understood the answers?
- What makes a good doctor/nurse/dentist?
- What would they change to make going to the doctor/dentist/nurse a better/more enjoyable experience?

The vignettes, story boards and picture cards were used with some groups more than others and, in particular, a more free discussion was encouraged where the children showed no interest in the vignettes or they were not considered age-appropriate. Where children wanted to tell a particular story or describe a particular experience, they were encouraged to do so. While every effort was made to engage with the children on all of the above issues, this was not always possible since priority was given in all cases, but particularly with young children, to keep discussions short (20-30 minutes) to prevent the children getting bored.

Interviews with parents

Nine interviews were held with a total of 30 parents, including two individual interviews and two interviews with both parents of the same child. The interviews were semi-structured in nature and aimed to gather evidence on parents' experiences of attending a range of health professionals with their children. While the issues discussed with parents mirrored those raised with the children (see above), they also explored parents' attitudes to the relationship between health professionals and their children, and issues such as obtaining consent. The length of interviews with parents varied from 20 to 90 minutes, depending on the time available and the nature of parents' experiences.

Interviews with health professionals

Interviews with health professionals were semi-structured and in some cases individual interviews took place over the telephone. They were necessarily short and focused (approximately 15-20 minutes) and had two purposes:
- The interviews attempted to elucidate health professionals' awareness of the need and right of children to be listened to as part of the consultation process and to measure the extent to

which they implemented this in practice. Professionals were specifically asked to explain any methods or approaches used when dealing with children and to identify both best practice in the area and any obstacles or barriers to such communication.

- The interviews explored whether health professionals had received any training on communicating with children and whether they would value further training in this area.

The group interviews took longer (approximately 60 minutes each) and allowed the issues around communication with children to be explored in more detail. While the same two objectives were pursued in the group interviews, these also addressed different issues depending on the constituency of the professionals involved. For example, the interview with the staff of the children's unit compared their approach to their colleagues outside the unit, while the interns spoke about bridging the gap between theory and practice, and the professionals involved in education focused predominantly on matters of curriculum and training.

Data analysis

The interviews were all transcribed as soon as possible after they took place. They were transmitted directly to the Project Coordinator and access to them was limited to the research team. The transcripts of the interviews were read through carefully whereupon obvious themes began to emerge. Their views were then grouped under a number of headings and additional issues were also identified. Interviews with health professionals were taken separately and their views were also collated under various headings. Their views on the issue of education and training were grouped separately and analysed together with the material from the curriculum audit.

Ethical considerations

The research team gave serious and lengthy consideration to the ethical and practical issues involved in this research, with guidance being drawn from *Ethical Principles for Researching Vulnerable Groups* (Connolly, 2003). Because the research was conducted in the community rather than in a formal healthcare setting, there was no mechanism available for formal ethical approval at the time it was carried out. The research was guided by three ethical principles: that the research be conducted with integrity and professionalism; that the rights and dignity of all those involved or affected by the research be respected; and that the well-being of those taking part in the research be ensured as far as possible. These principles raised a number of practical issues, which were dealt with as follows.

Piloting the methodology

Professional and ethical standards require careful preparation for research of this kind. For this reason, once the interview plans were finalised, a pilot was run with four children between the ages of 5 and 14 to determine the validity of the approach and the reliability of the responses received. The pilot was deemed a success and no changes to the proposed interview schedules were required. The transcripts for the pilot were not included in the overall study.

Consent of participants

Respecting the rights and dignity of the participants required first and foremost that everyone offered their free and informed consent to participate in the study. Best practice demands that, when researching with children, the consent of both the child and his or her parent or guardian is required and that these decisions are based on a full appreciation of what the research is about, how it will be used and what is expected of the participants. In this regard, every person involved in the research received a jargon-free summary of its objectives and purpose, together with the contact details of the Project Coordinator to whom any questions, queries or problems could be addressed.

When interviewing the children, the researcher explained the research to them in age-appropriate language, including what she wanted to talk to them about, and then gave them the opportunity to leave if they were not happy to take part. She asked for the children's permission to record the interviews and gave them the opportunity to listen to their own voices on the data recorder. Before the interviews began, the children were given the opportunity to ask questions and it was explained fully to them that they would not be identifiable from the research, but that their views and words would be honestly represented. To this end, all interviews were recorded and transcribed verbatim.

Once verbal consent had been given, the children were asked to sign age-appropriate consent forms. All children signed these forms, at which time they were given a further opportunity to leave the room without having to give a reason. Apart from one child who left one group discussion for a while and then returned later, all children and young people participated fully and freely in the group and individual discussions. A similar procedure was followed for the adults who participated in the research.

Confidentiality

Confidentiality is a key ethical principle, central to the need to prevent the research causing any harm to those who have participated or who are affected by it. A number of measures were taken to protect the confidentiality of the participants in this study. First, every participant was assured that their confidentiality and anonymity would be respected and that they would not be identifiable from the material made publicly available through the report. Consent to the use of the data recorder was sought at the outset of each interview, access to the transcripts was limited exclusively to the research team and the tape was erased once transcribed. All participants were assured that no-one would be identifiable personally from the transcript. To this end, each of the transcripts was given a number and group interviews are identified as such. The parents were identified only as such; the health professionals were identified with reference to their occupation; and each of the children was given a pseudonym once their interview had been transcribed. This system was used to ensure that no quotes could be traced back to individual people.

Every effort has been made to report accurately what children, parents and health professionals said during the research. However, some of the quotations have been edited minimally to ensure clarity of meaning.

Issues of child protection

It was of the utmost priority during the research that no harm or upset should be caused to the children involved. This included protecting the confidentiality of things said by individual children in the interviews. Accordingly, the children were assured that their comments would not be shared with their parents or others, unless at their request. There was one exception to this — namely, if the children revealed child protection issues.

In this regard, the guidelines issued by the Department of Health and Children (1999), *Children First: National Guidelines for the Protection and Welfare of Children,* were circulated and discussed by the research team who agreed a course of action to follow if something untoward was suspected or disclosed during the course of the interviews with children and parents. In particular, a procedure was designed to take steps to protect the child by reporting the information giving rise to concern about the child's protection to the responsible adult, while both explaining the necessity for doing this to the child and at the same time reassuring them that they had done nothing wrong. In fact, nothing of this nature arose.

5 EXPERIENCES AND PERSPECTIVES OF CHILDREN

The primary aim of this research was to explore the extent to which children's voices are heard in the healthcare setting and one of its principal objectives, therefore, is to record the experiences of children in this area. This chapter recounts these experiences and presents children's perspectives on their interactions with health professionals. The discussion begins with a profile of the children involved; it then recounts children's experiences of dealing with health professionals; it goes on to examine the effectiveness of professionals' communication with children, looking at the extent to which children understand the information provided by health professionals. Finally, it reports children's accounts of what they consider to be best practice among health professionals, what they would consider the ideal characteristics of a health professional and what they would improve about their healthcare experience.

Since this chapter is directed towards giving a voice to the children interviewed, it is inevitably somewhat varied in tone and material. However, it is important to represent faithfully the views of the children as they were presented in the underlying research. Throughout the discussion, the children's own words are set out in italics and the interview number at which these quotations were recorded is given in each case, using the acronyms CGI (for Children Group Interview) and CII (for Child Individual Interview) for ease of reference.

Profile of children interviewed

Fifty-one children, between the ages of 5 and 14, were interviewed. Twelve of these children had existing or once-serious health conditions that required them to have ongoing contact with health professionals. The remaining 39 had no particular health conditions, which meant that their involvement with the healthcare setting was less extensive than the other 12 children and therefore possibly closer to the average or typical experience.

An aim of the research was to include the views of children from as broad a range of backgrounds as possible. To this end, 24 children came from a poor socio-economic background and a further 6 may be considered to be at risk of poverty or in need. The research also aimed at a broad geographical spread and to this end, the children came from Longford (12); Cork (11); Dundalk (12); Dublin (9); Waterford (6); and Limerick (1), and from a mixture of rural and urban settings. The children's ages were 5 years (3); 6 years (4); 7 years (4); 8 years (9); 9 years (6); 10 years (8); 11 years (7); 12 years (5); 13 years (3); and 14 years (2). There were 16 girls and 35 boys.

The children were interviewed individually or in groups, normally without their parents, although in some situations parents were present. Four children were interviewed individually, while others were interviewed in groups of 2 (1 group); 3 (2 groups); 4 (1 group); 5 (2 groups); 6 (3 groups); and 7 (1 group). Further details on the methodology are set out in Chapter 4.

Children's experiences of communication with health professionals

During the interviews, all children were asked about the kinds of circumstance in which they had encountered health professionals and then whether, when they visited a health professional, he or she spoke directly to them or to their mum or dad. Children expressed varying views in response, but a common reply was that the professional spoke to child and parent simultaneously. This was the particular experience of children who had visited specialist children's hospitals, who were more likely to describe the doctors as tending to talk to them and to their parents together than those visiting general hospitals where the interactions tended to be more directed towards the parents alone (CGI 10).

For example, one boy, aged 11, who had visited a children's hospital many times told us that the health professionals there talked to him and his parents together, which he liked (CII 7). This experience did not appear to be widespread, however, and other children described how their doctors did not speak directly to them. According to Roisín, aged 13, *'There was really only one doctor that talked to me on my own without my mum and dad'*, whereas *'If I go anywhere else the doctor will just talk to mum and dad'* (CGI 13). The same girl reported that she was treated differently in an American hospital, where the doctors and nurses *'would talk to you, straight to you, instead of to your parents'* (CGI 13). Another girl, aged 12, similarly spoke of her experience of visiting hospital for an X-ray, where she said that everyone spoke to her mother and not to her (CII 14). This was in line with the view expressed by the older children interviewed, who noted that their doctor spoke to their parents rather than to them on their visits (CGI 13). In such cases, the health professional tended simply to acknowledge the child's presence, as Judith, aged 7, explained: *'He [the doctor] spoke to mummy ... he said hello to me'* (CGI 5).

Children's experiences of consultation varied depending on the nature of their interaction and of the professional with whom they interacted. For children who had to have medical procedures, such as X-rays or injections, their interactions were primarily with doctors. Children gave a varied response to the question of whether they were prepared for procedures or offered explanations before receiving an injection, having an X-ray or a more serious intervention.

For example, Niall, aged 10, explained that the injection he was about to receive was only explained to him *'sometimes, but not really'* (CGI 12). Similarly, Brenda, aged 13, commented that the nurse who gave her her medicine never explained what it was for when administering it (CGI 13). One group of children who had a lot of contact with the system (principally in a specialist children's hospital) reported that their doctors and nurses asked them first before taking blood or carrying out a minor procedure, and always explained what they were doing beforehand. These children felt happy to object if they did not want the procedure and many felt that, in these circumstances, the doctor or nurse would listen to them (CGI 10).

Children who had had an X-ray reported varying experiences. Those whose X-rays or scans had been taken in a specialist children's hospital reported that the radiographer had explained to them what they were doing and showed them the X-ray or scan afterwards (CGI 10). For example, Trevor, aged 12, explained to us about his experience of having a CAT scan: *'They'd do it in sessions so ... they'd ask you to put your hand forward ... maybe they were putting a needle in, finding a vein or something, and they'd be saying do this ... be superman ... And they'd tell you what was happening'* (CGI 12). Afterwards, he was shown a copy of his scan (*'It was a copy of my head and it was all hollow'*) and he was clearly happy that the person who took the scan discussed it with him (CGI 12).

However, many children complained that the radiographer had not explained the procedure to them in advance. The response of Roisín, aged 13, was typical: *'They just said to stand still and there'd be a little flash and it would be done in a few seconds'* (CGI 13). Few children were offered the chance to see their X-ray when it was taken, although many said they would have liked this opportunity, to see what their insides looked like (CGI 6). As Emmet, aged 10, said: *'They should have been telling us what was going to happen'* (CGI 6). For some children, without these explanations, the experience was frightening (CGI 2).

While children gave less detailed information about their experiences visiting their dentists, they tended to respond positively and, in particular, highlighted that dentists spoke directly to them (CGI 6). Three teenagers described their experience of the dentist in very favourable terms. As Sandra, aged 14, put it: *'They are there laughing and talking away to you and ... they've their hand in your mouth and you can't talk at all'* (CGI 13). Most children found it comforting that their dentist talked a lot to them. As one boy, Cathal, aged 11, said: *'The dentist who was taking out my teeth, she was saying stuff to me, talking to me ... they're always trying to make you laugh and all that to distract you ... it sort of distracts you from the pain'* (CGI 12).

Other children were less positive about their visits to the dentist, which many of them associated with pain. One boy, Dermot, aged 13, complained: *'And they don't even say, hold on now, I'm going to pull this. They just go ... zump!'* (CGI 11). When asked what would make the visit to the dentist better, Trevor, aged 12, said: *'If the dentist were to explain [things] and you couldn't see all the tools they were going to use'* (CGI 12).

Children's experiences with members of the nursing profession were generally positive. Judith, aged 14, who had a nail removed, described how the nurse *'explained when she was taking off my nail ...*

that it would grow ... back' (CGI 6). Children who had visited specialist children's hospitals commonly described the nurses as *'friendly'* and *'nice'* (CGIs 10 and 11). One boy, Frank, aged 11, commented: *'They're always trying to make you laugh and all that to distract you'* (CGI 12). Similarly, according to Trevor, aged 12, nurses *'make you feel comfortable more than the doctors. The doctor is trying to get organised and the nurse is just there to help them and to sort of speak to the children about what's going to happen'* (CGI 12).

Many children responded positively to the question of whether nurses explained things to them when they were in hospital. In general, the children described the nurses as easier to understand than the doctors (CGI 4). Positive experiences with other health professionals were also recorded by the children interviewed. One girl, aged 12, reported how she loved attending her physiotherapist because she *'explains what's she doing and why'* (CII 14).

Overall, while they had clear ideas of the characteristics that each profession should have, many of the children interviewed appeared to appreciate the contrasting approaches of doctors, dentists and nurses to communicating with them.

How children felt about consultation

While some children were happy for the doctor to talk to their mum or dad, most felt that the doctor should speak to them either in addition to or instead of addressing their parent. For example, Judith, aged 7 (helped by Paul, aged 8), said: *'I think he [the doctor] should be talking to you ... not the mams and dads'* (CGI 6). This view was shared by other children. For example, one boy, aged 11, told a story about a visit to a dentist who had not consulted him, just spoke to his doctors in the children's hospital and to his parents. When asked how he felt, he said: *'It annoyed me badly ... They didn't ask me, [they] only asked the doctors in [the children's hospital] and ... my mum and dad'* (CII 7).

Therefore, most children appeared happiest with the situation where the health professional spoke directly to them. One boy, aged 10, said that this direct communication *'made me feel better'* (CII 8). Another boy. aged 11, who had spent a lot of time in a children's hospital, described the other children on the ward liking the doctors who, in his view, knew how to deal with or talk to children. As he explained: *'I think children wouldn't like if the doctors just ignored them and talked to their parents'* (CII 7). Another boy, Aidan, aged 9, described feeling that *'there was something really wrong with me'* when his doctor spoke to his parent and not to him (CGI 5). Susan, aged 10, in the same group, agreed. When asked how she would feel if her doctor spoke directly to her, Sandra, aged 14, replied: *'I would feel that he is talking to me and not my parents. He's not acting as if I wasn't there ... I would feel better that he was speaking to me'* (CGI 13).

Overall, then, children felt better about the experience and about themselves when health professionals included them in the conversation about their healthcare.

The impact of age

In addition to recognising that they are treated differently by children's specialists than by general health professionals, the older children interviewed also noted a difference in the way they were treated now compared with when they were younger. They observed that while before, their doctor tended to talk to their parent, now they are spoken to directly (CGI 11). For example, Sandra, aged 14, remarked: *'When I was younger ... I'd go to the doctor and the doctor wouldn't really acknowledge me at all. But now he does'* (CGI 13). A boy, aged 11, who had had a lot of contact with health professionals, described a similar experience: *'When I was really small ... I can remember they talked more to my mum and dad than to me ... But as I got older, they ... talked to all of us'* (CII 7).

In another reflection of this point, Aine, aged 12, described in positive terms her experience of returning to a hospital where she had received treatment some years before: *'The other day I was up [in the hospital] and ... I saw a load of nurses that I hadn't seen for a good few years and ... they all came up to me and acted as if they were my age, and we talked about all the things I do'* (CGI 11). This clearly had a positive impact on Aine and illustrates the importance to children's self-esteem of being consulted directly by their health professional.

Children's views on the importance of direct communication

Many of the children interviewed had a strong sense of the importance of health professionals talking directly to them and were able to explain why this was important based on their experiences. Some children felt that they, rather than their parents, were better placed to explain what was wrong with them to the doctor (CGI 5).

For example, Sandra, aged 14, recalled one visit to the doctor where he asked her mother: *'How do they [referring to her] feel now?'* Sandra's view was: *'They don't know how I feel ... if they are asking you, then **you** can answer the question fully'* (CGI 13). A similar view was expressed by Brenda, aged 13: *'When I went in, I had hayfever or something. And they were asking my mum what was wrong with me? What were my symptoms? They could have just asked me'* (CGI 13). Again, a boy, Trevor, aged 12, complained about the doctor asking his mother how he preferred his medication. As he explained: *'Sometimes it's easier if they ask you if you want it in tablet or in liquid'* (CGI 12).

Some children identified a relationship between being consulted by the health professional and being able to understand their situation. Aine, aged 12, said that communication is important because *'children want to understand if they're sick ... what's wrong with them and if what their doctor is going to do will help them'* (CGI 11). Geraldine, aged 10, felt that *'the child needs to know what's happening'* (CGI 11), while Roisín, aged 13, noted that *'Usually, when they talk to my parents it's ... what's going on? What's happening? I think that if they were talking to me, I'd understand a bit more about what was going on'* (CGI 13). One boy, Mark, aged 11, told us that the doctor should *'talk to you, like tell you what's wrong with you'.* Instead, he complained: *'All he [the doctor] does is talk to your mammy and write something down ... and we go to the dentist [chemist] and he gives us stuff'* (CGI 2).

For other children — for example, Catherine, aged 6 (CGI 11) — understanding what was about to happen was important to allay fear. Receiving direct explanations from the health professional was something which the children interviewed regularly identified with being prepared for what was to happen. John, aged 8, said that if doctors did not talk to children *'You wouldn't know what they are going to do and you could be afraid',* while another boy, aged 11, said *'You'd really like to know what's going on ... so it makes it less frightening'* (CII 7). Dermot, aged 13, noted: *'They start saying all these big long words ... the children don't really understand [and] it kind of frightens them a bit'* (CGI 11). In addition, children commented on how a doctor might appear frightening and thought it was important that doctors try not to look scary so that the children would not be afraid. As Trevor, aged 12, put it: *'If they are kind ... you kind of get distracted'* (CGI 12).

Building an ongoing rapport with their doctor also helps children to deal with their fears. For example, Joseph, aged 8, commented that *'if the doctors never talk to the children and the children never talk to the doctors, they'll never know them'* and he thought it was important to build up a friendship so that *'they can see the doctor again and say hi'* (CGI 10). Building relations would allay the child's fears, according to Joseph, because *'children who didn't get to know their doctors [whose doctors did not talk to them] might be scared of them'* (CGI 10).

A final factor identified by some children was the objection that not being informed about what was to happen would make them less likely to comply with the treatment proposed. While Cathal, aged 11, said it was important for doctors to *'see how they [children] feel ... if they don't want the operation'* (CGI 12), others suggested that they would object on a point of principle if the procedure was not explained adequately to them in advance (CII 7).

While children identified a range of reasons, as outlined above, why their doctors should communicate with them as well as their parents, it is important to note that children did not object to the involvement of their parents. Mary, aged 10, could see the importance of the doctor talking to her mother as well as to her, noting *'if the doctor just talks to us [children] and he doesn't tell your mum, then your mum won't know what to look for ... [when you're not well]'* (CGI 2). Similarly, Niall, aged 10, understood that in an emergency it might be quicker to talk directly to his mum rather than to him. In his case, he said: *' 'cause it was kind of an emergency so she had to get it done quickly'* (CGI 12).

Overall, children's experience of communication with health professionals was clearly mixed. Among the factors that impacted on communication were the level of specialist experience of the health professional and the age of the child. However, regardless of their experience to date, children were clear that they wanted the doctor to talk to them more than they currently did and expressed important, principled and practical reasons as to why this made more sense. Having established the importance of communication to children, the next section will look at the effectiveness of communication from the child's perspective.

The effectiveness of communication

Children's understanding of communication with health professionals

During the interviews, children were asked whether they understood health professionals' questions or explanations. The children's responses showed that their understanding varied significantly and appeared to depend on the approach of the individual health professional and the child's age and maturity. When asked whether they understood the language used by the health professional, a common response — such as that of Frank and Harry, both aged 11 (CGIs 12 and 5) — was that they understood some but not all of what was said.

There were also more extreme responses from children, who said they understood nothing or, alternatively, everything that was said. For example, one boy confessed to not understanding anything his doctor said *'because sometimes he talks double Dutch'* (CGI 6). Alternatively, another boy, aged 10, commented that his doctor (a consultant in a children's hospital) used only language that he could understand and as a result, he said *'I understood everything, every word that came out of his [mouth]'* (CII 8), although he admitted this was not the case when he was younger. There is thus evidence that the experiences of children differ depending on their age and maturity. Catherine, aged 6, for example, admitted that she understood what the doctor said to her only *'sometimes'* (CGI 11).

This also highlights the important role played by the individual health professional, whose approach may facilitate the child's understanding. For example, Paul, aged 8, said that he was able to understand his doctor, who was testing his eyes, because he explained to him what he was doing (CGI 6). Another boy, aged 11, explained that the surgery was not a frightening experience for him because *'they were really kind to me and they explained in a way that I could understand ... what they were going to do'* (CII 7).

All children clearly felt it was important that the doctor explained things to them in words that they could understand (CGI 6). Regardless of their level of understanding, many children confirmed that they wanted their doctor to explain things to them (more) directly.

Children's willingness to ask questions

One way in which to address deficiencies in children's understanding of information provided is through responses to questions. As explained in Chapter 2, provided they are in a supportive atmosphere, children will generally ask questions in order to make sense of information given to them. It is therefore essential, in order for information-based communication to work effectively, for children to feel that they can ask questions if they do not understand what their health professional is saying.

As part of the underlying research, we asked children about their willingness and ability to ask questions and, importantly, what kinds of factors made them unwilling to ask questions or engage with their health professionals in this way.

Many of the children interviewed responded that they were happy to ask their doctor questions if they were unsure what he or she was saying (CGI 12). One boy, aged 11, explained: *'Well, if I had any questions I would always say it to them [the health professional] or mum and dad. And if I said it to them, they'd always explain it to me in a way I'd understand'* (CII 7).

Other children showed a willingness to ask their doctor questions if there was something they did not understand (CGIs 5 and 12) and they appeared comfortable to ask either their parent or the health professional for more information (CGI 12). This was a feature of older children especially. A number of 12-13 year-olds noted that if they had questions, they felt able to speak to their doctors about them. As Aine, aged 12, said about her doctor: *'Before I'd leave, he'd ask if I had any questions and, if I did, he would answer them'* (CGI 11). When asked what she would do if a doctor used a word she did not understand, Aine said *'I'd ask him to explain what it means and maybe use a different word, a shorter word, to describe it'* (CGI 11). She explained further: *'Well, if he says you've got this infection, I'd ask him what is it and what it does. Can I fight the infection?'*

The confidence of these children in asking questions may be attributable to the fact that many of them had considerable experience of the healthcare setting. Their preparedness to ask questions may have arisen from their greater experience in this regard. It may also be related, to an extent, to the degree of experience of the health professionals with whom they interacted. It is more likely that children who had long-term experience in the healthcare system would interact with professionals who were more experienced in dealing with children.

While some children felt free to ask questions, this was not a universal experience and a number of children expressed reluctance to ask questions. Frank, aged 11, admitted that *'I wouldn't be so comfortable with asking all questions because they just usually ... get on with it'* (CGI 12). Similarly, a girl, aged 12, said that she did not feel able to ask a question because she was *'afraid that he [the doctor] would say something that would make her look stupid'* (CII 14). Other children said they would wait and ask their parents any questions rather than ask their doctor. As Brenda, aged 14, said: *'If they are talking to you, then you'd ask questions. But if they are talking to your mam and dad, you'd feel like you're butting in'* (CGI 13).

This was also the experience of Dermot, aged 13, who commented: *'But most of the time they focus on the parents when they are answering the questions. They wouldn't actually look at you'* (CGI 11). He continued, *'Say I ask, what does that mean, he'd start talking to the parent about it. He wouldn't look at me'*. Asked how that made him feel, Dermot said, *'a bit left out'*. Aine, aged 12, agreed, saying that *'It's like it's the parent who is in hospital and not you'*.

One of the most interesting aspects of these children's experiences is that they tend to be older children who express reluctance to ask questions. It may be that, as children get older, they become more conscious of any hint of a patronising or dismissive attitude on the part of the health professionals with whom they are dealing. For these children, it is their greater awareness and sensitivity that makes it more difficult for them to ask questions.

Children's ideal model for participation

We considered it important to supplement our understanding of best practice by asking children how *they* thought the process of children's participation in healthcare decisions should take place. The children interviewed identified a number of key aspects of best practice, outlined below.

Use of age-appropriate language and props

The importance of providing children with information in an accessible form was discussed in Chapters 1 and 2. Interviews with the children confirmed that these issues were important and relevant to them also. There are special challenges in making information accessible to children and young people, and the children interviewed for this research made a number of suggestions as to how health professionals could provide information to children in an accessible way.

The children recommended several ways in which doctors could improve their communication skills, including using age-appropriate language and props. Some children suggested that health professionals *'should know how to talk to children'* (CGI 6). Judith, aged 7, advised *'Don't tell them [the children] big words'* (CGI 6). Similarly, John, aged 9, commented that a good doctor *'tells them [children] so they understand things [in] words that they understand'* (CGI 5). Trevor, aged 12, also advised doctors dealing with children, *'Don't use big words like they are only children. They didn't [go] to college or anything'*. Frank, aged 11, and Niall, aged 10, agreed that doctors *'should learn different ways to explain things'* (CGI 12). More innovatively, Cathal, aged 11, thought doctors and nurses should learn more clown tricks to keep children amused (CGI 12).

Some children, particularly those who had a lot of experience of the healthcare system, highlighted situations in which they had found the use of child-appropriate language and terminology or the use of props to be very helpful. One boy, aged 11, told how the word 'Freddy' was used to describe a cannula or an IV, and explained that he thought this was a good idea because *'If you say "cannula", nobody would understand it. Not the kids. But if you said "Freddy", then they'd all be going, oh yeah. So, it helps them understand'* (CII 7). This boy also recalled the use of a teddy bear to show him what was going to happen during his heart surgery: *'They have the bear. The heart bear ... And ... if you put your hand up you can actually feel the heart. And they used to use that to show you what they were going to do. And they used to actually put a cannula on the bear ... to show you what they were going to do'* (CII 7).

It seems clear, therefore, that children respond well to the use of age-appropriate language, props and other devices to help health professionals to explain things to them. These devices were popular among children themselves and their use should be more widely encouraged.

Preparation for procedures
Children clearly preferred being prepared for what was going to happen. As Emmet, aged 10, commented, a good doctor should *'explain what they are going to do'* (CGI 6), whereas another boy, aged 11, said *'if you know what they are going to do, then I think you ... feel less scared'* (CII 7). Frank, aged 11, who had had nine teeth removed in hospital, said that: it was a frightening experience, but *'if they explain what is happening, it makes it a bit easier'* (CGI 12).

Children's definition of a good health professional
Children interviewed were asked what they thought were important characteristics of doctors, dentists and nurses. Their answers revealed a lot about their experiences of these different professions and also highlight the importance to them of being treated by health professionals that are good-humoured, sympathetic and speak to them in language they can understand.

Children of all ages readily identified the characteristics of a good doctor as one who spoke to them and explained things to them in language they could understand. For example, Larry, aged 8, described that a good experience at the doctor's was *'when they ask you stuff'* (CGI 6). Harry, aged 11, noted that a good doctor *'asks the children questions'*, while Emmet, aged 10, said a good doctor *'explains things to children, tells them what's wrong with them'* (CGI 6). Trevor, similarly, noted that a good doctor *'explains stuff to you'* (CGI 12).

The importance of a child-centred perspective was also identified as an important characteristic of a good nurse. One boy, aged 10, had a clear idea of what a nurse should be like, saying a nurse should *'know what a child would want in a situation. Say I'm going to have something like an injection, try to make sure to tell the parents to just [relax] the child or something and try to make it not hurt'* (CII 8).

Children also identified the importance of kindness on the part of their health professional. One boy, Aidan, aged 9, noted that a good doctor is one who is *'kind to you'* (CGI 5). A girl, aged 10, who had had a high level of contact with the health system, thought that doctors should be *'healthy'* and *'friendly'* (CII 8). Trevor, aged 12, also felt that a good doctor was *'someone that's funny, because our doctor is always cracking jokes'* (CGI 12). Cathal, aged 11, said a good doctor was *'someone who doesn't hurt you'* (CGI 12), while Cormac, also 11, said that he wanted a doctor to be *'understanding'* (CGI 10). Aine, aged 12, said a doctor should be *'kind and funny'* because *'you really don't want to be around a doctor who is quite serious and ... a bit angry and doesn't want to talk to children that much. You want a friendly doctor who wants to talk to children'* (CGI 11). Geraldine, aged 10, also thought that doctors should be *'friendly and kind'* (CGI 11), while Kate, aged 13, said that your doctor should be *'someone you can trust'* because *'you don't want anyone that you don't trust trying to look after you'* (CGI 11).

In contrast, Dermot, aged 13, complained about one doctor he had encountered: *'Well, it's not that he wasn't very nice. I'd say he was just tired ... he was ... looking down ... and wouldn't be looking at us and he was kind of mumbling. If you asked something, he'd snap at you'* (CGI 11). Cormac, aged 11, also complained about a doctor who was rude to him, which he did not like (CGI 10).

Finally, the health professional's physical appearance and the first impressions created are clearly important to children. As Dermot, aged 13, explained: *'Maybe if they didn't always wear a uniform or a suit ...'* because *'they look very serious'* (CGI 11). Other children agreed that this might be frightening, particularly for younger children.

What children would improve about their healthcare experience

Suggestions for the training of health professionals

In addition to profiling their ideal doctor, nurse or dentist, children also made some suggestions about how their healthcare experience could be improved. For example, when asked what advice they had for doctors and nurses, they recommended that they should *'talk to you about it'* (CGI 13). Similarly, when asked what nurses should learn in their training, Emmet, aged 10, replied that *'they should know how to talk to children'* (CGI 6).

Other children expressed the view that they would like more of a say in their healthcare decisions and that doctors should learn more about this in their training. For example, Cormac, aged 11, said that doctors should learn *'not to push children too far'* (CGI 10). As he explained (and the other boys in his group agreed), *'Sometimes you really don't have a choice on whether you want this or that'.* When asked what they wanted more say on, he said, *'The choice as in if ... you had to get a blood transplant or stay for the night'.* Similarly, John, aged 8, recommended that doctors should *'try to ask children, is it hurting or is it not'* (CGI 10). Children clearly want to be consulted through the procedure and not just before and after it is completed.

Some children also thought it would be a good idea to reward those patients who behave well (*'If they were really good and ... weren't ... distracting the doctors'*) by giving them stickers or sweets (CGI 10). Cormac, aged 11, also thought that doctors should *'give them [children] a little toy to play with or a book to read when they are getting an injection'* because, as John, aged 8, commented, *'Some clinics have no toys and everything would be like ouch! They'd be feeling everything'* since there are no distractions (CGI 10).

Child-friendly environment

The majority of recommendations made by the children interviewed related to making the environment in which they attend health professionals more child-friendly. Children were generally critical of the toys and other facilities available in doctors' surgeries and in hospital waiting areas. For example, Declan, aged 12, said he found it *'dead boring'* and all there was to do was *'read magazines, play with babyish toys'* (CGI 6). Similarly, Mark, aged 11, said there was nothing to do in the waiting areas, where it was *'really boring'* (CGI 2).

When asked what he would change, one boy, aged 10, said, *'I suppose make it something like a child ... play centre ... Make nice paintings on the walls and stuff'* (CII 8). This would be important, he said, because it would *'make a child feel a little better like'.* According to Tom, aged 10, *'There could be ... a room and ... a wee bit more space ... where the kids can go in and just play, like do art and stuff'* (CGI 2). As Aine, aged 12, explained, *'It would be good if they make the waiting rooms ... more colourful and maybe have stuff for children and older children to play with while they are waiting'* (CGI 11).

Many children agreed that babies and small children were well catered for in waiting areas, with blocks and lego, but felt that there was nothing for older children to play with in the waiting areas of doctors' surgeries or in hospital (CGI 12). Brenda, aged 13, commented: *'You're sitting there with nothing to do. And it's very hard for a child to sit still and to not be active'* (CGI 13). As Dermot, aged 13, explained: *'Sometimes there's little baby colouring books ... but there's nothing really there for teenagers'* (CGI 11). Aine, aged 12, noted that in the hospital she attended, *'they had like colouring stuff for children and not really much stuff for like my age'* (CGI 11). These children suggested that the waiting areas have television screens or CDs for young people to play, or play stations to play with, although they appreciated these might get stolen. Declan, aged 12, recommended that: *'Doctors' waiting rooms ... should have ... one pile of magazines for grown-ups and one pile of magazines for children ... There's all little baby toys ... and it's not only babies who go to doctors in [his town] and [yet] they have no 8, 9 and 10, 11 year-old toys'* (CGI 6).

Frank, aged 11, explained that it was important to cater for older children also because *'then you would feel more relaxed if you're playing something'* (CGI 12). Many children shared the view that there was little entertainment for older children to prevent them getting bored.

In contrast, children who had spent lots of time in the specialist children's hospitals liked the range of toys available there for them to play with. One group of boys, aged between 8 and 11, was particularly pleased that games consoles were available in one hospital. When asked what they would improve, however, they commented that more toys were needed for the waiting area. For example, Joseph, aged 8, said: *'Put more toys 'cause you'd be bored sitting there ... just waiting and waiting'* (CGI 10). This was echoed by children in other groups (CGI 4).

Of their experiences in hospital, children recommended that beds should be *'more comfy'* (Dermot, aged 13, Catherine, aged 6, and Geraldine, aged 10, all thought this) and *'not one that squeaks every time you turn over'* (CGI 11). They complained about the *'funny'* hospital smell and Dermot, aged 13, also complained that *'the air is really heavy. And I don't think you can open windows'* (CGI 11).

Older children (aged 12 and 13) commented that they did not want to share the ward with younger children who *'might want to watch Barney'*, *'would wake up at three in the morning'* (CGI 11) or where the decorations of Winnie the Pooh were for small children (CGI 11). More generally, they felt that the children's wards catered more for children and babies than for young people their age. They thought the idea of a teenage ward was *'brilliant'* and Dermot, aged 13, recommended that it should be *'decorated with teenage [things], not Barney curtains and Bob the Builder'* (CGI 11).

Some of the children could see the improvement in the hospital they attended. For example, Aine, aged 12, who had a transplant at a young age said: *'They're like the rooms have become different and they painted the walls, but because the playroom when I went first was just plain yellow and you could only get in the games and all during the day because they locked them up at night. But now they have like you get play specialists there they take them out and there's more stuff in the playroom now to play with and the walls are all colourful'* (CGI 11).

Clearly these improvements were supported by children, who equally felt that there was a lot more that could be done to improve their experience in hospital or at the doctor's surgery by simply taking their age into account.

Summary

The children interviewed for this research varied in age, gender, background and the level of contact they had had with the healthcare system. Yet, despite these variables, their views reflected a consistent identification of the importance of being heard by their health professionals and being provided with age-appropriate explanations and information to help them cope with the consultation and treatment process. Children's need to be understood, and to be treated with empathy, kindness and good humour during illness, is strikingly clear from the research. The children interviewed identified a range of reasons, both practical and principled, regarding why this was the case.

Children's experiences showed a variation in the extent to which their preferred model of participation was allowed. While it is not possible to reach definitive conclusions at this point, it does seem that children who have come into contact with specialists in children's health or those working in children's hospitals had more favourable experiences and that they were better informed and more involved in their healthcare decisions.

Children also made valuable suggestions regarding how their interactions with health professionals could be improved. While many of the children referred specifically to their 'doctor' in this regard, their recommendations — to undertake training with regard to effective communication with children and to use age-appropriate language and props — were directed at all health professionals, including nurses and dentists. Children's recommendations that general waiting areas be made more child-friendly, particularly for older children, are simple yet clearly worthy of attention.

6 EXPERIENCES AND PERSPECTIVES OF PARENTS

While the principal purpose of this research was to gather the experiences of children, individual and group interviews with parents also provide an interesting and important dimension to the subject being researched. Parents provided valuable information about their child's participation in healthcare and the obstacles that prevent children's active involvement. Furthermore, because the legal requirement for consent generally requires parental consent *(see Chapter 3)*, the way in which parents respond to their children's participation in healthcare decision-making has an important practical impact on the level of participation that can be achieved.

Profile of parents interviewed

Overall, 30 parents were interviewed, either as parents of the children interviewed or completely separate. Two parents were interviewed individually, two sets of both parents were also interviewed separately and the remaining parents were interviewed in groups of 8 (1 group), 5 (2 groups) and 3 (2 groups). Parents interviewed included the parents of children with particularly serious or long-term health problems, and others who had more general experience of accompanying their children to the GP, dentist and hospital as required. In addition, one group of parents interviewed was from the Traveller community and their views provide a particularly valuable insight into their children's treatment by health professionals. The vast majority of parents interviewed were mothers, but three fathers also participated.

In general, the interviews focused on gathering parents' experiences of attending health professionals with their children. As well as discussing details of the factual issue of the extent to which doctors and others spoke to their children, and the level of information imparted to the child either directly or indirectly, parents also gave their views as to the appropriateness of such approaches by health professionals. This raises the fundamental question of whether parents can actually impede children's participation in healthcare decision-making. A particularly important issue arising from the interviews is the tension that can exist between the parent and the health professional regarding the involvement of children in the consultation process. Disagreement on the amount of information children are given, how they are given it and by whom arose throughout discussions as particularly significant sources of conflict and anxiety.

The material gathered is presented here under the headings of:
- parents' experiences of the child's communication with health professionals;
- understanding communication with health professionals;
- child-friendly environment and equipment;
- training for health professionals.

Throughout the discussion, the parents' own words are set out in italics and the interview number at which these quotations were recorded is given in each case, using the acronyms PGI (for Parents Group Interview) and PII (for Parent Individual Interview) for ease of reference.

Parents' experiences of the child's communication with health professionals

Overall, parents interviewed appeared to be content with the level of communication that health professionals had with their children. They rarely criticised professionals who failed to communicate directly with their children or to provide them with relevant information. Instead, they were more likely to object to their own exclusion or marginalisation from the consultation or treatment process, where the professional had focused on their children, or to complain that the professional was giving their child too much information. Parents' understanding of their own right to be involved in the process was a dominant feature of many interviews, while their awareness of their child's right to be listened to was not always particularly prevalent.

Criticism of direct communication with children

Many parents interviewed appeared to agree with or acquiesce in their child's lack of direct or active involvement in the consultation process. For example, some parents commented that nursing and medical staff spoke to them in detail regarding specific medical treatments for their children and did not go into great detail about these with the children themselves. They did not appear to have any difficulty with this approach (PGI 6).

Moreover, a significant number of parents criticised health professionals who sought to communicate directly with their children. Some adopted this approach because of their apparent view that the child has no right to be involved, while others did so in order to protect their child from anxiety or distress. The latter approach was illustrated by the parent of a boy with heart problems, who felt it was inappropriate for the doctor to speak about his surgery in front of her son. In her view, it was better that the child did not hear the discussion at all and she described that, to this end, her husband sometimes took the child out of the room while she discussed his treatment with the surgeon (PGI 4). This decision appeared to be motivated by her concern that the child's ability to comprehend what was being said added to his anxiety in certain situations. This was supported by the father's view — that he understood best what was in his son's interests. He commented: *'It is probably hard for the doctors to say ... what level of comprehension they are dealing with in a child and I would say with [my son] that very early on he had a fairly good level of comprehension as to what was being said and so it ... could cause a degree of anxiety in him ... at times'* (PGI 4).

Parents were similarly reluctant to allow their children to go through certain procedures alone and expressed the view that their presence at the child's side during dental treatment, for example, would reassure the child and result in a more positive experience (PGI 6). Another parent explained how she was allowed to accompany her child during dental treatment only because she had continuously insisted on doing so (PGI 6). A further extreme example was represented by a mother's explanation that it was better for her to hold down her child so that the doctor or dentist could undertake the procedure to which the child objected (PGI 7). Another mother explained, with apparent guilt, how she had held down her daughter for the doctor to give her a vaccination injection, when her other daughter leapt on the doctor's back to protect her (PII 5).

For some parents, the health professional's decision to communicate directly with the child was understood as the parent's exclusion from the process. One mother described feeling marginalised when the doctor dealt directly with her child and not her, and expressed the view that the parent should be spoken to first to allow him or her to determine what information the child was given. As she explained: *'When they came into the room [to treat her daughter], they didn't tell me what was going on. I had to stop them and ask them had I no mouth or something that they couldn't ask me? ... They shouldn't just ... ask the child without letting the parent know what exactly they are doing'* (PGI 1).

Another parent thought it was more efficient to simply talk directly to the parents rather than to the child: *'By the time they are finished with the child and go on to the parents and then ask about the child, they are wasting a lot of time and I think that [they] might go directly to the parent'* (PGI 1).

Parents who criticised direct communication with children appeared to range from agreement or consent with their child's non-participation to a more formal objection to the child's direct involvement in the consultation or treatment process with the health professional. A commonly expressed view was that parents were better placed than health professionals to determine the level of consultation that was in their child's interests. In this way, some parents are acting as the gate-keeper to the child's exercise of his or her right to participate in the consultation process and would seem to be limiting the level of participation that may be achieved.

Parents' support for their child's involvement

In contrast, a smaller number of parents showed support for their child's participation in consultations or dialogue with health professionals. These parents favoured the professional communicating directly with their child and providing him or her directly with relevant information. An approach favoured by one parent was where the nurse would explain the process to her, but do so by including her son: *'[The nurses would] show you what they're doing and what they are going to do with the child ... They'd explain [it] to me, but they'd be looking at him when they are telling me, which is letting him know what they are going to do'* (PGI 7).

Other parents showed an awareness of the importance of the child's direct communication with the health professional. As one mother explained, where a doctor fails to speak directly to the child, *'That's leaving the child out then. And then the child feels that as well'* (PGI 1).

Another mother, herself a nurse, felt it was important for her 10-year-old daughter that the doctor focus on her, given that she was capable of articulating how she felt and explaining this to her doctor (PII 5). The mother described as *'wholly positive'* an experience of attending her GP, where the doctor conducted the consultation process entirely with her daughter because, as she explained, *'her daughter was the best person to answer her doctor's questions as she knows best'.* While she took a back seat during the consultation, she was reassured in the process by the fact that the doctor maintained brief eye contact with her, particularly when writing the prescription. This mother recalled a similarly positive experience with regard to the orthodontist, where her daughter went in alone for her consultation and then she was called in afterwards (PII 5).

It is apparent from the research, therefore, that parents have a strong role to play in supporting the child to communicate directly with their doctor. This is clearly a conscious decision on the part of some parents. As one parent said: *'When we go [to the hospital] we encourage him to ... ask the doctor about it. I suppose we've kind of forced him to get involved himself'* (PGI 4).

Parents' behaviour can be decisive as to whether their child is listened to by the health professional or is a silent bystander in the consultation process. The attitude of health professionals was also identified as a factor, however. One woman criticised her doctor's approach in this regard when she described bringing her 13-year-old daughter to his surgery: *'He won't ask her ... he'll ask me what way is she complaining? What's wrong or what's her problem? ... I would explain it the best I can ... but ... she is 13 years of age ...'* (PGI 1).

Overall, therefore, a range of factors can be seen to inform whether the parent takes up the role of a supportive intermediary, who facilitates communication between the child and the health professional, or whether the parent dominates the consultation process by presenting a barrier to effective communication between the professional and the child. Interviews with parents illustrate that factors such as the capacity for direct communication with the health professional, as well as the parents' perception of whether the child is capable, play a strong role here.

In this regard, some parents saw their child's evolving capacity as an important factor to take into account in facilitating or promoting his or her greater involvement in the consultation process. Parents expressed the view that their child was old and mature enough to enjoy direct communication or involvement with the health professional. Parents also noted the difference in treatment in their child as he or she got older and recognised the importance of his or her evolving capacity to be involved in the consultation process.

For example, the mother of an 11-year-old boy, who had had ongoing medical treatment, explained: *'We're coming through a changing process ourselves ... at the moment. [Our son] is getting older ... now ... 65 or 70% of the time [the doctor] focuses on talking to [our son] ... So he's talking to us through [our son], but he's directing the conversation to [him] and then we get an opportunity to ask questions ... I think personally that's about the right balance, you know ... I don't like to see a situation where they deal with [him] on his own, but definitely knowing the type of child [he] is, I think that I'm happy with the mix we're having at the moment, [where] we're ... spoken to through him, [where] the focus is on him by the doctor'* (PGI 4).

The boy's father shared this view, noting that soon the child will want full independence. As he noted: *'In another two years ... he won't want us to come into the room with him ... Now he may not still have a choice about that ... but you can see him ... taking a lot more control of it. And, I mean, at 18 he has all the control at that point anyway, which isn't so far away, you know'* (PGI 4).

This case illustrates how parents whose children have had ongoing contact with the healthcare system are well placed to evaluate their child's evolving capacity to be involved in the consultation process. It may also highlight the fact that health professionals who build up a rapport with child patients over a long period of time are well positioned to take their evolving capacity into account and modify their style of communication accordingly.

Preparing the child for procedures

In discussing the importance of children's participation in the healthcare process, some parents, particularly parents whose children had had surgery, identified the child's need to be prepared for the process. One mother described a distressing experience, where her child was being prepared for surgery: *'In [my son's] case ... they put an oxygen mask up to his face and he went ballistic and he backed himself into a corner ... I remember the Sister on the ward, the doctors, everybody came in and they were all standing there trying to get him calm. He was like a caged animal. And the Sister ... said, we're getting nowhere with him, back off. And he got back into bed and he lay down and he came around himself ... she certainly listened to him'* (PGI 4).

Children themselves have identified the importance of being prepared for the procedure that was about to happen to them *(see Chapter 5)*. The above quote dramatically illustrates this point, while also showing the importance of listening to children in this situation. While the issue of legal consent does not arise here, the importance of preparing a child for a procedure or surgery is important from practical and emotional perspectives. The impact of this lack of preparation on the child's recovery from surgery was also identified here: *'He had his surgery when he was six and he was brought in as an emergency ... It was a nightmare for him because he wasn't prepared and there was a huge difference between his recovery, his response, his whole stay in hospital was very traumatic as a result of not being prepared for it'* (PGI 4).

In this context, parents interviewed understood clearly the importance of their child being provided with the necessary information, both for medical and emotional reasons. As one mother explained: *'They feel so powerless ... Because ... if you say to them, "You're going to get blood taken and it's going to hurt, but it will end after a few minutes", they're more likely to let you do it, than if you say ... "Sit there and I'll tell you a story" and next thing they're taking the arm off them'* (PGI 4).

The importance of building a relationship of trust with the child before carrying out even a minor procedure is clear, therefore, and is worthy of greater research.

Showing empathy with sick children

Parents criticised health professionals for sometimes failing to have empathy with a sick child. As one mother put it: *'I think sometimes, maybe, they forget that the kids are sick and they're miserable, they want to be left alone. They don't understand, especially the smaller ones, ... why they are there and they have to be given leeway ... and ... some amount of control about what's happening to them'* (PGI 4).

Parents also distinguished between different doctors, identifying some as more child-friendly than others. For some, the contrast could be seen within a specialist children's hospital, where it could not be presumed that all specialists were child-friendly. As one mother, with extensive experience of such a hospital, put it: *'You know, there's one doctor ... who's absolutely fabulous and he's great with the medicine ... but he doesn't even look at the child ... he doesn't even see the child. And the same with the surgeons: they don't see because their field is different'* (PGI 4).

However, the contrast could also be seen between the children's hospital, where professionals were perceived to have a child-friendly approach, and the general hospitals, where this approach was not always evident. The same mother as above continued: *'Suddenly when you come outside [the children's hospital], it's completely different ... No matter who you come across, they don't treat children the way they do in [the specialist children's hospital]. I think ... on the whole, the majority of people in [the children's hospital] accept that this is all about children, but outside of that I don't think they do'* (PGI 4).

The view of parents was that the health professional who related well to children was not necessarily the person who had chosen to specialise in children's health or was attached to a children's hospital. This echoed the view of children, who felt it related to personality rather than to profession. This further strengthens the case for the provision of formal training in this area.

Understanding communication with health professionals

The extent to which children understood communication with health professionals arose in interviews with parents. However, the use of comprehensible language and providing adequate explanations were important issues from the parents' perspective also. This was especially evident in responses from Traveller parents and from parents from a socially disadvantaged background.

Use of elaborate language for explanations

Several parents, particularly those from the Traveller community, raised the issues of language and literacy as communication barriers. This affects both children and their parents, as one woman explained: *'I think if they are training they should know there is a language barrier between Travellers, and these are Traveller children, and doctors do come out with big words, not just to children. Like even when I go in to see the doctor, it is very hard to understand'* (PGI 2). Another woman described what she saw as unnecessary use of complicated language, explaining: *'What's stopping them from using plain simple words? ... I don't understand why they can't use easier words'* (PGI 1).

For these women, the doctor's failure to explain the situation to them was a more obvious problem than the failure to explain it to their child. As one woman said: *'The doctor wouldn't tell you what's wrong with the child; [he'll] just ... sign over the medication and give it to you'* (PGI 1).

However, for many parents, the doctor's failure to explain things to them has a knock-on effect on the child. Like the children interviewed, these parents explained how fear can arise as a result of the lack of understanding. As one parent said: *'Half the time it's frightening mammy and daddy, not to mind the children'* (PGI 2). Another parent felt that the fact that children may not understand what the health professional is saying meant that parents have to spend a lot of time explaining things to them (PGI 2).

In addition to the fear generated by the lack of effective communication with health professionals, some parents described how the failure to communicate effectively can have more serious consequences. As one woman described it: *'They'd ask you questions like "Is your child allergic to anything?" But if your child wasn't on medication, you don't know if they are allergic or not, so that's still not explaining things'* (PGI 1). Another complained about the lack of explanation on the vaccinations her child received, saying: *'But they didn't tell me what all the vaccinations were for. They just said ... she will have to get this, never said for what reason'* (PGI 1).

Overall, it is clear from the interviews with some parents that the failure to provide adequate explanations of the child's condition and the prescribed remedy affected the quality of both the parent's and the child's experience with the health professional. Thus, the use of complicated language as well as the failure to take time to provide adequate explanations to parents were identified as clear barriers to effective communication about their child's health. As with the children, this inability to understand created unnecessary fear among parents and could be said to impede the development of a relationship of trust between parent and health professional.

However, for some Traveller women who had had many negative experiences of health professionals, this contrasted with their positive experience of public health nurses. As one woman explained: *'I think the only one that has time for the children is probably the public health nurse when she comes around. She gives you more time ... because she'd sit down and she'd listen to your problem and about your child and ... you can explain everything to her'* (PGI 1).

Use of written literature for explanations

Literacy problems among the Traveller population also mean that the failure of either doctor or pharmacist to explain medication to them may have serious consequences. As a Community Group Facilitator explained: *'Travellers' reading and writing skills aren't very good and ... "Take two 5ml spoonfuls three times a day" makes absolutely no sense ... it's a spoon in the morning, a spoon in the evening'.* But as the parent explained, *'You don't know the dose, the shape and size of the spoons'* (PGI 1).

According to the Facilitator, this problem extends beyond the Traveller community and affects everyone with literacy problems: *'In Ireland a quarter of the population has literacy problems and I just don't think that health professionals dwell on that enough. They feel they are covered if they give out the literature, but that would be like ... giving out literature in French to everybody ... I think I have a responsibility if I was giving a drug to somebody that they should know how to follow the instructions'* (PGI 1).

Child-friendly environment and equipment

The need to treat children in a child-friendly environment was raised consistently by both parents and children interviewed for this research. The contrast between the child-friendly conditions and equipment in children's hospitals and general hospitals can be seen in a number of different areas. For example, the failure to adapt the waiting environment or the diagnostic equipment was raised as a problem by several parents. Some parents felt that the equipment, like X-ray machines, should be adapted for smaller children, to make it easier for parents and children alike. One mother described the difficulty she encountered when her baby, who could not yet stand, needed an X-ray. She recommended that *'with the smaller children, the younger children ... they should have different equipment or ways of putting them sitting'* (PGI 1).

Several parents shared the view that child-friendly machines should be made available and that X-ray rooms, if not machines, could be made more child-friendly. One woman expressed her view as follows: *'They should [make] the X-ray room ... more cheerful looking and maybe their favourite kind of cartoon ... maybe if they were standing up, you could have the child standing up alongside it'* (PGI 1). Another woman agreed, saying there should be ways of encouraging children while they are waiting, say, for an X-ray. One mother felt that this was time that could be better spent preparing the child for the procedure to come. She explained that because children might be afraid on seeing the big X-ray machines, there should be *'things ... for children that [explain] — this is good, you have to do this, this is really good — encouraging them on'* (PGI 1).

Without these supports, many parents described the difficulty and stress involved in having to spend long periods waiting for small children to be seen by health professionals. Parents found it a particular challenge to occupy their children for long periods when waiting for hospital appointments or to be seen in the A&E room. As one woman described the situation: *'In casualty ... you've got to wait to be seen ... There should be a playroom to occupy their mind ... children would be depressed because they're bored'* (PGI 1). Similarly, many parents recommended that more be done (including providing more toys) to make the long waiting period easier for them and their children (PGI 7).

Parents also felt that children should not be kept waiting in hospital casualty areas, where they were unable to protect their children from seeing people injured in serious accidents or from drunk patients particularly at night (PGI 7). Some parents felt that children should be given priority in such cases.

Training for health professionals

Parents identified the need for greater training as the key to enhancing the level of communication between children and health professionals. On the issue of training, one mother said: *'A lot of the time they don't even look at the child, the doctor talks to parents ... and there's no consideration given to the child at all. So ... that's a huge [issue], especially for doctors, that has ... to change if they are going to deal with children'* (PGI 4). For this mother, training was the difference between her child's positive and negative experiences: *'Certainly when we would have gone with [my son] when he wasn't prepared as opposed to when he was prepared, or people that weren't nice to him, you know that makes a huge difference'* (PGI 4).

Another group of parents agreed, saying that: *'They'd want to give them training [on] how to communicate ... with children, how to deal with children. Or if children were sick, how to get through to them ... Just getting to know them'* (PGI 1). Another parent commented that it seemed to make a difference whether the doctor had children or not. As she put it: *'I think if doctors have children themselves, they seem to have a lot more ability to manage children, to deal with children and talk to children. So the training [is] through their life experience rather than through their education'* (PGI 1).

Another parent recommended that a person be assigned a liaison role — one whose *'total 100% focus is liaison between family, medical staff and child'* — to fill this gap and ensure that the valuable time of medical professionals is not taken up with non-medical duties (PGI 4). Others felt that nurses had a role to play in improving communication between child, parent and health professional. For example, strongly echoing the views of children themselves, one woman described the importance of the nurse being good-humoured with the child: *'When the child comes in, they should laugh and try and play with the child ... and let them know that [hospital] is not a bad place to be. Some of the nurses ... are fierce snappy and that doesn't help the child when they're going to be seen by this person afterwards'* (PGI 1). Another woman added: *'They should stop and be friendly. I think for all nurses and doctors, especially, they should be friendly ... they shouldn't be so serious with them'* (PGI 1).

A woman from a Traveller background identified the need to make doctors accessible to Traveller children. As she explained: *'Most Travellers are not as well educated as doctors are ... Children are frightened going in to doctors 'cause some children might never have been there before, so if they had pictures of all different cultures and hung up Traveller pictures ... they'd know it was for everyone'* (PGI 2).

Summary

The views of parents on their experience of attending health professionals with their children are rich and varied. It is perhaps simplistic to conclude that the views of those with a high level of contact with the healthcare system (such as those whose children have long-term and serious health problems) show a greater awareness of the importance of their child's participation in the consultation and treatment processes. However, on the basis of these interviews, greater involvement with the health professional does seem to impact on parental views on participation.

A range of factors clearly affect the parents' views of the child's capacity and readiness to be fully involved in any communication with health professionals, not least the parents' own understanding of the process and of the right of their child to participate in it. An important issue identified in the interviews is the conflict that can arise between the parent and the health professional regarding the process of consulting and informing the child about their health and healthcare. The fact that parents who did not appreciate health professionals' attempts to involve their child directly in the process were motivated by a variety of reasons — ranging from a lack of awareness of the child's need and right to be involved, to the need to protect the child from unnecessary anxiety — demonstrates the complexity of this issue. It also highlights the importance of raising awareness among parents about the child's right to be heard and the need to ensure that health professionals receive the necessary skills and training on how to communicate with both parents and children in this setting.

At the same time, parents' identification of the need to adapt the hospital environment for children is entirely consistent with children's own views *(see Chapter 5)*, as is their recommendation that health professionals need to show greater empathy with their child patients, to build relations with them based on trust and to communicate more directly with them. The need to provide training for health professionals in this area is also entirely consistent with the recommendation of children and the health professionals themselves.

7 EXPERIENCES AND PERSPECTIVES OF HEALTH PROFESSIONALS

The views of health professionals regarding children's participation in healthcare decisions constitute an essential aspect of this report. During the research, individual and group interviews took place with a number of health professionals with a view to identifying their approaches to communicating with children and to exploring their experiences and attitudes in this area. While this discussion focuses on professionals' experiences in practice, details of their training and education are set out in Chapter 8.

Profile of health professionals interviewed

The aim of speaking to health professionals was to understand their perspective in relation to communicating with children in the healthcare setting. To this end, individual interviews were carried out with 22 professionals with experience of children's healthcare in the community and in hospital, including general practitioners (GPs), dentists and nurses, specialists in children's healthcare (such as children's nurses, paediatric consultants and play specialists) and specialists in other areas (such as anaesthetists and ENT consultants). In addition, three group interviews were carried out — with the (mainly nursing) staff of a children's unit in a general hospital; with a group of hospital interns, also in a general hospital; and with tutors, lecturers and professors involved in the education and training of a range of health professionals, who had come together to discuss the teaching of communication skills. In all, 50 health professionals were interviewed for this research project.

This mix of health professionals ensured that the research benefited both from the particular experience and knowledge of those with specialist expertise in the area (e.g. children's nurses), those at the start of their medical careers (i.e. hospital interns) and those with responsibility for the education and teaching of health professionals.

While the number of professionals interviewed (50) is a relatively small sample of those working in the healthcare setting in Ireland, the research is enriched by their breadth of experience, the different levels of contact they have with child patients, the different purposes this contact must serve and the many other factors that may affect the nature and quality of that interaction. This, together with the variety in approach and background among interviewees, means that the material provides a useful snapshot of the experience of some health professionals in communicating with children. It is not without its limits, however. In particular, it is likely that professionals who agreed to be interviewed for this kind of project have already acknowledged the importance of children's participation at some level. For this reason, therefore, more comprehensive research is recommended relating to the participation of, and more general response to, children in the healthcare setting from the professional's perspective.

The material gathered is presented here under the headings of:
* health professionals' strategies for communicating with children;
* obstacles to communicating with children;
* attitude and approach of parents;
* the issue of a child's consent to an intervention;
* awareness of best or bad practice;
* attitudes towards education and training.

As will be seen from the following discussion, many of the health professionals have developed sophisticated and thoughtful approaches to communicating with children and show a clear understanding of the need to do this. However, this tends to occur in an individualised way and there seems to be little opportunity for professionals to share their experiences or views. Moreover, it does not always conform to the best practice identified in Chapter 1 of this report.

Throughout the discussion, the health professionals' own words are set out in italics and the interview number at which these quotations were recorded is given in each case, using the acronyms HPGI (for Health Professionals Group Interview) and HPII (for Health Professional Individual Interview) for ease of reference.

Health professionals' strategies for communicating with children

Many professionals interviewed were reluctant to identify any one approach that they took when communicating with children, describing their practice as individualised. For example, a dermatologist explained as follows: *'It really depends on the child and each consultation is very much individually tailored. And it depends what the child is like when they come into the consultation room. You get some children who are very open, you get others who are hiding behind their parents' legs. So it depends on what the child is like. And a lot of the time I would start by talking to the parents and … the child would be sitting on their parent's knee, depending on what age they are … I don't have a set way of doing it'* (HPII 4).

Similarly, an ENT surgeon explained that he had no single approach, but tried to treat each patient individually. He also explained that he would *'try and communicate … the basics of what's happening, what's wrong with them … what we are going to do about it, in as much as it's possible'* (HPII 12).

Many health professionals favoured an approach that varied depending on the child's age and maturity. These and others described a variety of techniques for communicating with children, including relating to them and to their parents and respecting their physical boundaries, using age-appropriate language and props, showing empathy and building trust with them.

An important aspect to be taken into account in developing strategies to facilitate the communication process relates to the objective of the interaction and the level of urgency involved. For example, it is not possible to equate the approach taken in a busy A&E room with that provided by a long-term care team. However, as will be seen below, strategies can be employed in both situations which are appropriate and yet which take account of the child's right to participate in the decision-making process.

Taking account of the objective of the interaction

Clearly, not all health professionals have the same amount of time to spend with a child; nor do all consultations meet the same needs. Some professionals, like social workers, psychologists and play specialists, may see a child a number of times, enabling a particular style of communication to be adopted. For these professionals, their ongoing interactions offer the opportunity to develop more long-term strategies to deal with patients. A paediatric social worker explained her approach as follows: *'I would be very much non-directive in terms of letting the information and the conversation … be veered very much by the child. I'm not going to force them to talk about things they're not comfortable with'* (HPII 1).

A psychologist in a similar position explained the diversity of approaches that she uses to communicate with children: *'We would work a lot through art. I would … do a lot of drawings … Or sometimes we'd play games while we're talking … The less articulate children are always a challenge, whether it's through anxiety or through lack of ability or speech problems … but we would also do a lot of play therapy, things with dolls and … with medical techniques or medical conditions we would try to explain them through drawings or through dolls … and we'd have a lot of medical equipment that we can show them how things are done and let them role-play that with dolls'* (HPII 3).

This psychologist also explained how she approaches such consultations: *'When they come in, we tend to ask them do they know what a psychologist is? Why they're coming? And maybe give them an idea of some of the things that we would … see usually, including their own possible problem. And I suppose with that age group [5 to 14 years] usually they seem to be generally quite happy. Of course, there's always the very anxious child, who is anxious about everything, and that takes quite a bit of skill'* (HPII 3).

These different perspectives illustrate the approaches used by health professionals who have a longer timescale to work with the child and/or who address more deep-rooted problems. Where fear is known to be an issue, as with dentists, a paediatric dentist explained how this was addressed: *'First we would find out what that fear is based on, you know … Was it the white coat? Was it the*

57

smell? Had they a previous bad experience? So, first we try and get as much information as possible ... some cases would be quite difficult if the child was very uncooperative, so first of all we would have an assessment with them, what their fear is based on and if we can work around it' (HPII 22).

In contrast, health professionals who have just a short time to elucidate important information from a child, as in an emergency, have to take a slightly different approach. For example, an A&E doctor explained her approach as follows: 'When we're planning the treatment, we tell them what we're planning to do. We're usually very honest with them. So, we give them the information and ... we'd supplement it to the parents if they needed it, but most would be centred around the child when they come in to us. It's all verbal communication that we use really' (HPII 6).

Similarly, an anaesthetist explained that he needed to take a direct approach: 'I ask a whole series of questions and I am fairly direct about those and I won't answer any questions casually or informally while I'm getting my information. I'll actually interrupt questions to say "I promise I won't leave your bedside or leave here until I've answered all your questions, but I need to ask questions first of all" ' (HPII 16).

Inevitably, time constraints mean different levels of communication and participation depending on the circumstances. The important point, however, is that appropriate strategies must be employed for the circumstances involved which retain a commitment to the ideal of communication with and participation by the children.

Talking to children or their parents

Many of the health professionals interviewed explained that they spoke to parents first, instead of talking to the child. They explained that this was important where the child was of a young age or in order to elucidate certain important information. Like some of the parents interviewed, an intern recognised that it was simply quicker, in some circumstances, to talk to the parent. She explained: 'The child is there because [the parent] brought them to the doctor, the child didn't go themselves. So, they can tell you what their concern is ... there are only so many hours in the day and they are more likely to know why they're there' (HPGI 2).

However, a more common response among interviewees was to adopt an approach that varied depending on the age of the child. This could involve direct or indirect communication with the child, perhaps via a parent. An anaesthetist explained his approach as follows: 'If they're ... 7 or 8 upwards, I like to talk to the child rather than the parents. I mean you really are talking to the parents because obviously the child cannot give you the answers you want really. But ... I do try and ... look at the child and make them feel that they're the ones I'm dealing with, which I am of course ... But if they are 5, I have to say I talk to the parents because that's too young really to reasonably expect to engage a child at that stage' (HPII 15).

An ENT surgeon explained that he adopted a similar age-appropriate approach as follows: 'Usually ... most of the questions are directed towards the parent. Usually it depends on their age ... We're talking to the child and the parent, but obviously most of the questions are to the parent. Then, over a certain age ... we'd question the child directly ... ask them why they are here? What their problems are?' (HPII 12).

An oncology consultant explained that at the initial consultation his enquiries 'may well go through the parents or may well go through the child. The older child I would address directly in the presence of parents, but the younger child ... I would obviously go through the parents' (HPII 23).

Understanding the child's capacity

Given the extent to which health professionals stated their preference for an age-appropriate approach, this raises the issue of whether the professional in question is well positioned to determine the capacity of children to understand or be directly involved (see also Chapter 2). One factor that is important in this context is a professional's awareness of the child's development. A paediatric dentist explained: 'I mean, the most important thing is ... the child's development ... at what stage their learning capabilities are at, and directing appropriate learning capabilities to that because I think it's important that, if you are dealing with children, everyone should know ... what can a 5-year-old cope with? What can a 5-year-old understand and [equally] 12-year-olds?' (HPII 22).

A nurse manager also explained the importance for professionals to be aware of a child's development and what he or she can rationalise at different stages. She explained how with *'a 7-year-old, you can sit down and talk to them. The majority of them you can rationalise with ... because they will understand. Once you've got to know them and they are happy with you, they'll come round. [But with 2-year-olds] ... all you can do is a small amount of play with them; you cannot rationalise with them'* (HPGI 1).

A social worker also highlighted the importance of those who need to communicate with children in a medical setting to have *'a good understanding of children's development, or how children operate'* (HPII 10).

However, the issue of what developmental stage an individual child has reached and the extent to which health professionals use this factor to choose which approach to take was not raised consistently in interviews. Child development aside, professionals acknowledged the relevance of the age of their patient. As one nurse explained: *'For the 5-year-old to, say, about 6, sometimes 7, depending on the child, you would use very friendly terms, keep the air nice and light, your approach is very open and friendly with them so they don't feel intimidated by what you're about to do'* (HPII 13).

Interviews highlighted that health professionals who are not used to dealing with children might not understand the reason for their behaviour during treatment. As a clinical nurse specialist explained: *'Sometimes it could be behavioural problems that they have. And that's what you have to be careful about. That it may be a behavioural problem that the child has and that you have to be able to recognise that, that it's not just pure boldness or it's not just fear of me and that they can't actually handle it'* (HPGI 1). She explained that those in other hospital departments may not be able to see these problems and may misinterpret them: *'... the fact that people down in A&E ... are not used to seeing how we deal with the behaviour we see, so they automatically take this child as uncooperative and that the parents have no control'* (HPGI 1).

This highlights the need for raising awareness of child development and psychology among all health professionals, as well as offering training in children's health to every professional likely to deal with children, not just child specialists.

Relating to children and respecting their physical boundaries

One GP explained her approach as one which attempts to relate to children. She described a consultation as follows: *'You would do a combination of things: speak to the mother, it's more often the mother, and to the child. It depends on their age. If they're 11, I would stand outside my desk and we would chat and I would generally break the ice with them, talk to them about different sorts of things. What class they are in at school? What school they were in? Holidays, whatever it happens to be, Halloween, that sort of thing. And then ask them a history of themselves if that's appropriate. That would be about it really'* (HPII 2).

Another GP agreed that the approach varied from child to child. She explained the importance of reading body language, saying: *'I would be aware of, for example, not separating the child from the parent and therefore threatening it. So, the child would always be allowed sit beside the parent or on the parent's lap if it wished. If the child was obviously feeling more confident in the room, it would probably have moved away from the parent and would be playing with the toys, in which case I would actually get down on my knees and move over to the child and maybe start talking to the child about some neutral topic, like the toy they are playing with, and play with them for a while and stay with neutral topics for a while'* (HPII 5). Moving on to the verbal communication, she explained: *'If it was an older child, maybe ask them about their friends, their favourite TV programme, what games they like playing and stuff. And then, when I felt that the child was gaining in confidence and maybe feeling more comfortable, you can move into the specifics.'*

As this quote demonstrates, this GP had a clear understanding of the importance of physical behaviour or body language when consulting with children. This was echoed by others. For example, an intern explained: *'I think sitting down ... really helps patients react differently in the bed when you sit down and talk to them. When you're standing, it's like you're just ready to leave in a minute'* (HPGI 2). Another intern explained the need to *'read'* the child's body language to determine whether the child is afraid: *'I always try to make sure the child is following me. You can sense it when the child — in probably a non-verbal response, a facial expression, how they look at you — whether they are ... scared'* (HPII 2).

An anaesthetist explained the need not to invade a child's personal space. He explained: *'I ... don't try and get too close to them either, as I think most kids don't like you being too near them'* (HPII 15).

Clearly, body language and non-verbal communication play an important role in the communication between child and health professional. Professionals' awareness of this can affect the nature and success of their interaction.

Age-appropriate language and props

While many health professionals chose to direct technical or medical questions to parents, others showed an awareness of the need to simplify technical language so that children could also understand. One anaesthetist described his dual approach: *'Most of the sort of questions that have technical words in them I'd ask of the parents, like anyone in the family with allergies, any medication your child is taking at the moment. But I direct to the child a certain number of questions. Always the following: "Have you any loose teeth?" and then I say the words "any wiggley ones" and "Have you had a runny nose or snuffles or sniffles?" and direct that to the kids'* (HPII 16).

Others showed an awareness that language may impede their communication with the child, although they were not specific as to how such a problem could be tackled. One GP, who described language as an obstacle to effective communication with children, explained the need to try to find ways around her use of language and children's lack of knowledge of the language she might use (HPII 2). As another GP explained: *'Obviously, as an adult, your world is different from the child's, you don't know what their language is'* (HPII 5).

In this regard, an oncology nurse explained how she used age-appropriate language, for example, when taking blood from a child: *'You would just say, "I'm going to go take some ribena from you, from your Freddy"* instead of saying blood (HPII 10).

The use of emotion cards was also highlighted by those working in A&E departments and by interns as a useful way to communicate with children regarding the amount of pain they are experiencing (HPGI 2). As one A&E doctor explained: *'If we're trying to get a pain score from them, we have a visual analogue scale, which is just a row of faces getting sadder or happier, whichever they feel'* (HPII 6). Others also described using visual aids. For example, an intern described using drawings to explain things to a child: *'I do drawings sometimes, especially if [they] are having trouble [understanding] ... they often wonder what's going to happen. Even for bloods, [it] means nothing to a child, but we explain, you know, [how it will] make them breathe better'* (HPGI 2).

A clinical nurse specialist described the importance of showing children what they were going to do, using props if necessary: *'If we were putting a catheter into a patient, you'd show them a port, you might even go and get another patient who has a port and let them see it. Or you'd show them a picture of what it would look like in another patient. You'd go and get an X-ray of somebody else and show them, "This is what it looks like on an X-ray" ... Most of our ... kids ...like to look at their X-rays; they want to know where the heart is, where the lungs are'* (HPGI 1).

For younger children, a play specialist may be engaged in order to facilitate communication and to alleviate children's fears. A play specialist interviewed described the nature of her role as follows: *'A child that comes in through A&E is very traumatised, first time in hospital. So the nurses would call me out and I would introduce myself and provide immediate play suitable for the child's age and stage'* (HPII 8).

As described in Chapter 5, the children interviewed for this research valued these attempts to involve them and to assist them in understanding the procedures involved.

Empathy with child patients

Both children and parents clearly identified the need for health professionals to empathise with children. This need was recognised by health professionals also. As an intern explained: *'I think it's true that we sometimes lose sight that there's a child in it, because you're just very focused on getting your job done and the parent gives you the story surgically anyway'* (HPII 2).

As a play specialist explained, children's attitudes are different and this must be borne in mind when treating them. She explained their attitude: *'Once it's over, it's generally over and they're not worrying about the next event, next week or the week after. They very much live for now and for the present. You'd see them recovering from surgery ... they're out of hospital much quicker, say, than an adult who would go in for similar surgery. Because if they want to get up and mobilise after their surgery, they'll just get out of bed and go to the playroom'* (HPII 1).

Clearly, some understanding of children's attitudes and perspectives is important to ensure effective communication with them by health professionals.

Building trust

A social worker explained the need to build trust with children and to communicate with them at their level. As she explained: *'You need to be able to establish a good rapport with them and you need to be able to develop trust with them and to develop open communication with them'* (HPII 10). The importance of honesty in communicating with children was also stressed by other health professionals. For example, a paediatric dentist noted that *'we find that you should never lie to a child'* (HPII 22).

A paediatric dermatologist described the need to build trust as follows: *'The parents usually give the story and tell the problem and then we will examine them [the child] and, obviously, you have to engage with them because first of all they are not going to undress easily unless they like you and that. So we would usually have some preliminary conversations with them to relax them. And ... then we ask them their permission, "Is it all right to examine you?" and they're usually ... fine. There would be a few who wouldn't be ... and then we work around that'* (HPII 17).

A clinical nurse specialist explained the importance of dealing honestly with children: *'If the child asks me something, I will always be truthful. Now ... you have to gloss it up or whatever, but ... I would not lie to them because I can't. If I tell them a lie and they're seeing me every single day, they're not going to trust me'* (HPGI 1).

Interviewees recognised, however, that building up trust can be a luxury in some circumstances because it takes time. A clinical nurse specialist explained the important role of the play specialist in this context, who could be engaged to deal with a child who is upset. She explained one scenario: *'We actually involved [the play specialist] and we used to bring her [the child patient] up to the playgroup ... she was terrified ... eventually over time ... she associated coming in with the playgroup and then we gradually brought her down to the clinic and she'd come down afterwards to the clinic and we'd see her here. Now she's fantastic, we've no problems at all. So, for some children, it [involving the play specialist] can be very helpful'* (HPGI 1).

One paediatric dentist explained that, in their profession, dentists must be particularly aware of the invasive nature of their practice. As he explained: *'Because everything we do is invasive ... the mouth is so sensitive we have to be very careful. We just have to use certain wording around certain things, so rather than saying an injection we'll say we're going to wash the tooth. So we change the wording slightly and show them as much as we can. We try to keep it as interactive as possible'* (HPII 22). For this reason, also, this dentist explained that it was important that children retain a sense of control. He encourages this as follows: *'I'll always say to them, if you want me to stop at any point lift up your hand, so they feel they are part of the treatment as well. So, if they want me to stop for a rest or anything like that, then I stop straight away'* (HPII 22).

Giving children choices

Many health professionals described the importance of giving children choices as to how the treatment can proceed. As a paediatric dentist explained: *'They can have an option of doing it* under local anaesthetic, sedation or a general anaesthetic ... so, depending on their fear or [vulnerability], we'll decide on which treatment we'd go for' (HPII 22).

Similarly, an anaesthetist described giving his child patients a choice by saying to them: ' "There are two ways to go to sleep for your procedure tomorrow: one is to blow into a balloon and you'll go to sleep slowly over about 3 or 4 minutes and it's a little bit like a space mask ... Or the other option is to get a pinch on the back of your hand", and I actually take their hand in mine and give it a small pinch' (HPII 16).

Nurses also explained that it was important to present children with a choice, however limited that might appear. A children's nurse explained that this works as follows: 'The choice isn't about whether they get treatment or not. The bloods must be done. [It's a question of] what way would you like it done?' (HPGI 1). Other options given to the child included 'Would you rather somebody read you a story?' and 'Or do you want to sit on your mother's lap?'

Offering children choices is clearly consistent with making their participation in the process of their own care meaningful and reflects the wishes of the children themselves, as identified in Chapter 5.

Explanations and preparation for procedures

Like the interviews with children and parents, many health professionals also identified as very important the need to explain things to children and to prepare them adequately for procedures. An oncology nurse explained the best practice in her area as follows: 'You'd sit down and show them, or if they are going for a scan, say there are books here of photographs of what the X-ray machines are like, or if they are going for radiotherapy the same approach ... so it's a multidisciplinary approach to communicating with children. There are doctors, nurses, we've got a ward psychologist and so ... everybody has an input into communicating' (HPII 19).

Similarly, a paediatric dentist explained his approach as follows: 'You have to show them everything ... one of the main things we called "Tell, show and do", and what that basically means is that you tell a child what you are going to do, show them it and then you do it' (HPII 22).

Asking questions

Some health professionals explained how they felt it was important that the children ask any questions they might have. As a paediatric dermatologist explained: 'I'll often say at the end, "Johnny, is there anything you wanted to ask me?" And you really do have to probe a bit because they could be having a terrible time of it at school. They could be bullied in school or whatever, and it wouldn't necessarily come out ... So one has to be very sensitive to that and I think in dermatology, in particular, you have to be sensitive to how, if you look different from your peers, you are going to be at risk of ... being teased and bullied' (HPII 17).

However, as one child psychologist explained, it was not always easy to get children to ask questions. She explained that in her work in a children's hospital: 'A lot of my job is ... to get them to ask the right questions or to ask any questions of the consultants or even to get them to ask the junior doctors ... Some of the doctors are excellent at explaining things to them if only they [the children] would ask. But a lot of doctors don't offer information unless you actually request it' (HPII 3).

An intern also explained how he would give the child certain information only if prompted to do so by the child asking questions: 'It depends if the child asks me a question. I will answer a question. If the child is 10 or 11, I would definitely answer the question. But I ... might not be as overt as I would be with the parents' (HPGI 2). This shows clearly how important it is that children are encouraged to ask questions and to participate in the decision.

It is clear from these examples that there is a great deal of good practice among health professionals. However, the benefits of this may not be fully maximised. Ways must be found to mainstream this knowledge through training and informal networking.

Obstacles to communicating with children

Many professionals interviewed were able to point to obstacles that prevented them from communicating more effectively with their child patients. These included a lack of education or training; lack of resources; the physical environment in which they work; the pressure of time; and the lack of a shared approach by colleagues. The attitude and approach of parents was also identified as an obstacle by some health professionals — an issue which is dealt with separately below in order to reflect its importance.

Education or training

While not all professionals identified the lack of education or training as a specific barrier to communicating with children, some highlighted the relevance of their experience in this area. For example, a children's nurse expressed the view that confidence in one's approach was important when relating to children: *'The other thing, from the point of view of communication, is your own personal confidence and knowledge ... and your own ability to translate it to the appropriate age group. To simplify it and to assess quickly ... how much can this child take on board now, today, first visit ... If you don't fully understand what you're talking about or perhaps, you feel the person is going to ask you a question and you don't have any knowledge of it, it's going to completely affect your communication ... if it goes badly between a doctor and a patient or a nurse with the patient, maybe it's because that individual didn't pick up on it or didn't have enough information'* (HPGI 2).

Resources

Some professionals expressed the view that the system within which they work and the resources to which they have access restrict their ability to employ some techniques that they might otherwise regard as best practice. As one ENT consultant put it: *'I would be aware, for example, of the Great Ormond Street style, where people very much communicate directly to the kids ... I looked at that, and again I would find it quite difficult [because] ... we don't have a paediatric hospital [or] a paediatric set-up here and it's somewhat difficult [to implement in practice]'* (HPII 11).

Physical environment

The lack of proper space to engage in meaningful consultation with children was identified as a clear barrier to effective communication by many health professionals. As a paediatric social worker explained: *'Here, in this hospital, we have no space to effectively communicate with children. If I'm meeting with a teenager or ... a young child on their own to talk about whatever has come up ... if I can't talk to them in the ward on their own because of their mother or other people around, I'd bring them to the surgical rooms, the treatment rooms. We're clambering over chairs, they're dull lifeless rooms ... it's not enticing at all'* (HPGI 1).

A paediatric dermatologist highlighted the lack of privacy as a particular problem in this context: *'You are in a room where there are students, there are the consultants, the junior doctors, nurses, parents, buggies, and you're trying to examine them behind a flimsy enough curtain and all sorts of people walking in and out of that room with records and things like that'* (HPII 17). Interns also explained the lack of physical consultation space as follows: *'There's not much [room] really for that in hospitals because the rooms where you can take somebody aside and talk to them quietly ... are hard to find ... it's usually a corridor'* (HPGI 2).

Nurses also complained about this problem, with the impact of this on the quality of care being explained by a nurse manager: *'If you want to raise the morale of a child, discuss something with parents, if you have nowhere private to bring them to discuss issues with them or to do therapeutic play. It may not be appropriate to do it at the child's bedside because maybe you may want to remove them from the environment that they are in and take them to a safe place'* (HPGI 1).

In addition to the lack of space, the lack of a child-friendly environment was also identified as a barrier. As one dermatologist explained: *'In some of our out-patient settings, they are not dedicated paediatric settings so we don't have child-friendly furniture and we don't have readily available toys and play things for the children to occupy them. So ... that would be an obstacle and I think we should ... have dedicated children's clinics'* (HPII 4).

A GP described the importance of having in place a completely child-friendly environment. The ideal situation, according to her, might be: *'The receptionist would have been chosen because they would have been child-friendly. The waiting room would have toys in it so that it would be child-friendly.*

When they would come into the room, the room was organised so that, for example, things like sharp bins and that sort of stuff were out of reach, so that you're not continually interrupting, saying don't touch that or whatever. There would be toys on the floor so the room is child-friendly' (HPII 5).

This was noted to be important in the A&E area of a hospital also. As one nurse manager explained: *'It's not an appropriate environment to have children in A&E and out-patients, where perhaps people are coming in behaving anti-socially, and you're putting them in a threatening environment'* (HPGI 1).

Time

Time was also identified by health professionals as a clear barrier to communicating with children. One GP explained that it was difficult to adopt an ideal approach within a limited timescale. An A&E doctor shared this view, saying that time was an obstacle *'because, by its very nature, when you're working in emergency medicine you have to see them [children] fairly quickly and you don't have an awful lot of time to spend with them. So it's obviously quite direct'* (HPII 6).

An ENT surgeon agreed, saying: *'To ... communicate with children properly ... it requires a reasonable amount of time ... Sometimes you've 60 patients sitting outside the door, so I would say subconsciously time is one of [the barriers to effective communication]'* (HPII 11).

A nurse manager at a children's hospital also explained how difficult it is to communicate effectively with children given the pressure of time. She explained that health professionals have to balance this with treating the child quickly: *'If a child is unwell, you want to get things done fairly quickly for them and so sometimes communication can fall down because you want to organise a test or a procedure, and maybe the child isn't fully informed or prepared for that procedure, and maybe the parent knows everything and doesn't want them to know ... and suddenly it's all happening together'* (HPII 20).

As one paediatric social worker explained: *'There's a lack of consciousness sometimes about small listening ears and about leaving information that's going on in front of children and ... you worry about news being discussed in front of children and just complete unawareness of the effect of that and the damage that can do'* (HPGI 1).

Lack of a common approach

Many professionals, particularly those who have specialised in children's healthcare, raised the lack of a common approach among colleagues as a barrier to ensuring that children are always treated in a manner consistent with best practice. Some expressed the view that poor awareness and understanding of the importance of communicating with children meant that children are not always dealt with in a consistent manner in a hospital setting.

Children's specialists in children's hospitals also recognised the need for all health professionals to adopt a common approach. As an oncology nurse working in a children's hospital explained: *'Working alongside other nursing staff ... it's very imperative that we're all singing from the same hymn sheet ... that one person doesn't do their own thing, that we're all adhering to the same protocol, that we're all doing the same thing'* (HPII 13).

Health professionals working in the children's unit of a general hospital also expressed considerable frustration at the lack of understanding of children in other areas of the hospital where they also have to be treated. In particular, children's nurses explained that it was not uncommon to have spent time building a relationship of trust with a child, only to have that destroyed by the intervention of another health professional. One nurse manager explained: *'You could spend some time winning confidence, having a child who is consenting, quite happily, to have an injection or procedure done and usually that is the start of this relationship and it can be undone in a flash by a third party coming in saying the wrong thing. Saying "Come on, hurry up, I have you now, hold out your arm straight, you're not doing it straight", just enough to turn everything back to square one'* (HPGI 1).

The failure of health professionals to adopt a common approach thus leads to problems. The same nurse manager as above explained: *'... where you have a doctor and a nurse or two nurses — one has established the relationship with the child and has gained their consent and is getting places. The second person comes in and suddenly comes in at a different level of communication with the child and the child is confused. Two people dealing with them in two completely different ways'* (HPGI 1).

To avoid this, health professionals proposed the establishment of a shared approach, as well as consistent training for all health professionals. They also recommended the agreement of protocols between health professionals to deal with practical situations, such as where one professional takes the lead and the other assists quietly, without getting involved actively with the child. This requires understanding, throughout the healthcare profession, that *'children communicate on a one-to-one very well'* and this must be borne in mind when teams deal with children in a hospital setting.

Attitude and approach of parents

From the perspective of health professionals, the role, attitude and approach of parents is frequently decisive in determining the nature and outcome of the consultation and treatment processes involving children. While the attitude and approach of parents was widely identified by health professionals as a barrier to effective communication with and successful treatment of child patients, it is clear that it can also be a positive influence on the health professionals' experience with the child. Regardless, it is clear that the dynamic between children, their parents and health professionals represents a challenge for all parties engaged in the healthcare of children. This is also reflected from the parents' perspective in Chapter 6.

One GP articulated the challenge for health professionals in communicating with the child in the presence of a parent as follows: *'It's one of those difficult consultations in the sense that ... the parent is the patient by proxy almost, and you end up communicating a lot with the parents'* (HPII 2).

While some children complained that health professionals spoke first to parents and then to them, and some parents complained about health professionals who marginalised them by speaking directly to their children, many professionals interviewed also recognised the important role that parents play. One GP suggested that there was a strategic reason for talking to parents before talking to the child: *'I would start by talking to the parents and getting them at their ease because I would feel, if they are at their ease, the child would sense that and would therefore be more receptive'* (HPII 5).

Difficulties posed by parents for the communication process came from a number of sources. Some professionals felt that the fears of parents can be transposed onto their children unwittingly and that this made the process of communication more difficult. As a paediatric dentist explained: *'If the parents have grown up with a fear, then the child ... will definitely have that fear as well ... even if the child hadn't experienced anything at all'* (HPII 22). An anaesthetist shared a similar view regarding the level of anxiety that is put on children by their parents: *'If the parents are uptight, invariably the kids will pick that up very quickly. And all of those are obstacles to making the whole thing ... as pleasant and manageable for the kids as possible'* (HPII 16). An oncology nurse working in a children's hospital also shared this view: *'If you've got a highly anxious parent, nine times out of ten you've a highly anxious child because they are taking their cue from their parents'* (HPII 13).

Professionals also described a reluctance on the part of parents to have their children know that they had a serious condition. A paediatric oncologist explained: *'When you have parents who come up here for investigation and we discover their child has cancer, the problem we often face is the reluctance on the part of parents to allow us to inform the child'* (HPII 23). An intern also expressed this perspective, in slightly different terms: *'I think sometimes the client doesn't want you to kind of say too much in front [of the child] ... I've often got the impression that I'm kind of rushing through it, so I don't say anything that might upset a child'* (HPGI 2).

Other professionals explained how parents sometimes tell their children too much. As one clinical nurse specialist described: *'Then you have the other extreme, where you have parents who, we think, tell far too much to their children and there's too much openness and everything is said in front of the children, which is in some cases, I think, not always good because you can put too much responsibility on them. And I don't think in some cases they're able for it'* (HPGI 1).

A GP identified parental attitude as the greatest barrier that she perceived to communicating with children. As she explained: *'If the parent has a positive attitude coming to the doctor, a good expectation of what would happen when they bring the child to the doctor, that consultation with the child is usually good as well. When you have a problematic relationship with the parent in terms of health-seeking behaviour or helplessness, or over-medicalising things, whatever it happens to be, you run into more problems with the child'* (HPII 2).

A radiographer also explained that *'parents are inclined ... to interfere slightly'* and this can have a negative impact on the consultation or treatment. In particular, saying that the child is likely to have difficulty with a procedure, the parents may actually cause the difficulty to arise. As the radiographer explained: *'Sometimes they'd make the child more nervous. They walk in and say, "I don't think she's going to stay quiet for you now" and I kind of say, "Well, sure I think she looks like a very good girl who is going to stay very still for this X-ray", and you're trying to tell them not to say that, because it makes the child behave like that, you know'* (HPII 18).

A staff nurse in a children's unit of a general hospital identified the same problem, describing it as *'disastrous'* where *'if you're going in to do bloods or something and the parents say, "They're not going to cooperate, they're not going to do it", you know ...'* (HPGI 1). An ENT surgeon gave a similar example of the negative influence parents can have on the communication process: *'We sometimes have parents who have preconceived ideas like, for instance, I had a child recently who was in for an operation and the parent said, "We've told the child they had to come to have their photograph taken" (nod, nod, wink, wink), wanting me to take part in the process. And that's obviously a bit disconcerting for everybody and then, of course, the child becomes hysterical when they find they're in the hospital. So a lot depends, I suppose, on the parent'* (HPII 12).

While some health professionals saw some parents as a barrier in the communication process, it is significant that other professionals did not recognise parents as an explicit barrier to communication with their children and instead described their role in this context as a natural one. As an anaesthetist explained: *'I certainly wouldn't see parents as a barrier. I don't think you can deal with a child of that age without the parents really being part of it ... They are still a family and I know children are individuals, [but] I think they see their parents as pretty central to their lives and ... I have no problem having parents there at interviews. They are probably helpful if anything'* (HPII 15).

Moreover, the importance of having parents present was highlighted by an anaesthetist, who explained the dilemma in his area as follows: *'The whole business of separation is extremely important and the practical issue that faces us all the time is whether or not we should separate child from parent prior to the actual induction of anaesthesia. And there are pros and cons ... But it's an extremely important one because some kids will remember being taken from their parents, say, in a holding area or reception area and will remember that as a very unpleasant thing. The other side of that is if a parent is brought into the operating theatre where they sort of help with the inductions and the child is asleep or very nearly asleep by the time the parent leaves. Then, in essence, the operating theatre team are dealing with two patients rather than one, in that the parent becomes the second patient. So, those are the two sides of the argument and practice varies or is split between those two. I think communication might be the key to solving that one'* (HPII 16).

Another anaesthetist explained: *'For many years, there has been a controversy ... from an anaesthetics, surgical and nursing point of view as to whether parents should be present at induction ... for elective paediatric cases over the age of 18 months ... I would regard the presence of the parent to be of benefit rather than the opposite'* (HPII 21).

Anaesthetists were not alone in sharing this view. A haematology nurse also explained how she felt that parents had a right to be involved and to determine the approach taken: *'You can only tell a child as much as a parent allows you to tell them and if they ask you to please don't mention it or please don't tell them, then you have to respect that'* (HPII 19). Similarly, a nurse manager shared this view, saying: *'They [parents] often wouldn't want to leave their child alone to have any conversation with any member of the healthcare team ... As health professionals we have agreed [to] try to work through why it is they may not want to tell a child something and try [to] work with that* and respect their wishes ... For the parents I want to make sure that the conversation that I'm having, that they are happy for the child to hear and because I'm very aware that children who have got chronic illness are very perceptive and have been through a lot more than children who haven't' (HPII 20).

Professionals' strategies for dealing with parents

Professionals recounted a number of strategies for dealing with parents who want to limit the information provided to their children. A paediatric oncologist explained the approaches he employs, which involve 'informing the parent of the diagnosis first and asking them to talk to their child where the child is young, or alternatively where the child is over 10 or 11 years informing them that the news is bad and giving them a choice as to whether to hear full details with or without their parents' (HPII 23).

Similarly, an oncology nurse explained her approach to highly anxious parents in such circumstances: 'We would say to the parents: Yes, we appreciate this is a very upsetting and traumatic time for you; however, for us to be able to do what we do best for your child ... I need [you to] work alongside us and any fears ... you have ... don't portray them in front of the child, so that ... they don't see ...that mum and dad get all anxious when they see a medical person or nursing member coming to them' (HPII 13).

Issue of child's consent to an intervention

The discussion so far has concentrated on health professionals in their communications with children. However, a core issue that remains to be addressed relates to the issue of consent. As noted in Chapter 3, while parents may give a legal consent to a medical intervention on behalf of their children, the child also has rights in this regard. In particular, the imposition of treatment on a resistant child raises issues relating to the protection of the child's rights of autonomy, dignity and bodily integrity.

Many of the health professionals interviewed explained that it was necessary to talk to a child's parents in order to obtain consent for a surgical or other procedure. However, others explained that the reality of dealing with children was that consent must be obtained from them also before intervening. A nurse manager explained how children 'won't consent to allow you to do some things', whereas a clinical nurse specialist put it thus, 'In general I think one thing about children — you won't do something unless they want it. That's as simple as that' (HPGI 1).

For specialists in children's healthcare, the issue of gaining the child's agreement and assent to a procedure was vital to its success. Imposing a procedure on an unwilling child raised an issue of assault in some cases. As one nurse manager explained: 'When is it right or not right? When does it become assault? If a child really doesn't want something done and you feel it has to be done and the child's objecting and the parents aren't saying anything, you're in a very dangerous area' (HPGI 1).

Children's nurses clearly articulated the futility of forcing children to have procedures done. This was also connected with the lack of a common approach between professionals working in children's healthcare (see above). As one children's nurse explained: 'The one thing I think people have to learn is, you try bloods twice and, if you don't get them, you get out and I think nurses should say that to the doctors — "Out, enough". Once you start going the third or fourth time, you're getting extremely frustrated ... and I think, as nurses, we have to say to the registrar or the SHOs [Senior House Officers] or whoever is taking it, "That's it, out" ' (HPGI 1).

Similarly, a nurse manager explained the impact that proceeding in such cases can have on the child: 'If the child is really objecting and he's very sick and we're there doing bloods or, say, passing a nasal gastric tube down their nose or whatever. And they're objecting, you're not getting anywhere ... you've got no consent, the child is screaming, you've got to think, long-term, are you providing this child with the most horrific memory that's going to keep them awake every night for the next six months? That's wrong' (HPGI 1). An alternative approach advocated in such circumstances was, for example, 'to bring the children out of the room for a while and let you go and play with them or ask [the play specialist] if she's around in the playroom to come in and give them a break' (HPGI 1).

However, children's nurses explained that it can be difficult to intervene to stop a doctor in these circumstances. Experience and confidence were both vital characteristics in this context. As a nurse manager explained: *'It takes a while but, ten years ago, if I was in a room with a doctor and he was doing blood four times ... I wouldn't have said no, sorry, enough. And now I know I can say no, sorry, and I'm well within my rights as a nurse within that team to say this isn't right'* (HPGI 1). Similarly, a children's nurse explained how she had to develop the confidence to intervene in such circumstances with some doctors: *'It might be just a matter of pride with them; they don't find a vein and they don't ... admit defeat that they didn't get a vein or seem to be not good at taking blood or whatever'* (HPGI 1).

This is clearly an important issue, worthy of far greater attention that can be afforded to it here. In particular, research into the development of joint protocols among health professionals should be undertaken to ensure a common and consistent approach is adopted and children treated in accordance with the highest standards. This recommendation is consistent with those raised by health professionals themselves, who supported greater multidisciplinarity and the sharing of common approaches to the treatment of and consultation with children (HPIIs 1 and 10).

Awareness of best or bad practice

As mentioned in Chapter 1, there are clear standards for best practice in this area. Responses of health professionals to questions regarding their awareness of best practice varied from one individual to another, as well as from area to area. Many interviewees did not appear familiar with any established best practice or written guidelines in their profession on how best to communicate with children. Moreover, some professionals questioned the relevance of best practice, describing what they did as *'common sense'* and *'derived from experience'*.

As one anaesthetist explained: *'I don't make out that what we're doing is any big deal ... there's no point trying to. You don't want to frighten them, you know. But I think it's one of those things; if you've been at it a long time, I think you just naturally, by trial and error, eventually come to a technique that seems not to alarm people too much and works most of the time. I mean, there's always the exception, but I don't think you can ever be right every time ... You have a lot of variables there ...you've got the child, you've got the parents and you've got the doctor, and each one has a different personality and what would suit my approach ... might not suit another person ... I think it is extremely difficult to come up with ... a way to say this is the best way to approach a child, you know. And every child is different as well. And, as I say, when you've analysed it there is infinite variability between the three different partners in the interview ... I think you've got to go with your own personality too. I mean, I'm sure other people do it differently to me and I'm sure they are just as good at it, but it's just the way I do it and it kind of works for me, I suppose'* (HPII 15).

A GP held a similar view. While she was aware of clear guidelines, she found they were *'quite impractical in the day-to-day situation'* and would have quite a number of limitations. She was, overall, *'aware of what best practice is'*, but *'very sceptical about the whole concept of best practice'* (HPII 5).

Nevertheless, several professionals, including interns, referred to the good or bad practice that they had witnessed during their clinical training or education. For example, a child psychologist remembered male trainees who adopted teasing behaviour with children, which a lecturer had pointed out was an *'aggressive'* way of relating to children. This example of *'bad practice'* had remained with her as a result (HPII 17).

One intern described a negative experience where the health professional/team leader was *'cold, short, fairly blunt'*. The intern went on to describe the impact of this behaviour on the rest of the team: *'When you are there and you know ... that everyone in that room is petrified and they don't really know what is going on and they're probably just too scared or too anxious to go ... further. I've rarely been in that situation, but I can remember one time when I was and ... it was just terrible'* (HPGI 2). For the family, the intern explained, the impact of this negative experience was also obvious because of the relationship between the patient and the health professional. She explained as follows: '... *because ... patients look up to the health professionals to kind of help them along with things and explain things properly and to be supportive, but sometimes I think that that can kind of get a bit lost, and maybe doctors more than nurses end up just giving the information and just leaving the patient with it, without anything else*' (HPGI 2).

The role of clinical education in developing best practice is discussed further in Chapter 8.

Education and training

It is evident from the preceding discussion that professionals have limited awareness of formal best practice in this area, although many of them would appear to adhere to best practice in the approach they take. As noted earlier, the professionals inclined to participate in this kind of study are more likely to have a higher level of consciousness of the issues involved. In this context, the question of education and training for the broader healthcare community arises.

Many health professionals — notably but not exclusively those who were trained as specialists in children's healthcare — expressed the strong need for everyone dealing with children to have paediatric training. One dermatologist explained the differences in approach between children's specialists and specialists in other areas: '*If you look at the difference between a paediatrician dealing with a child and a person who is not a paediatrician, there is a stark contrast*' (HPII 4).

Similarly, an anaesthetist explained how he relied on nurses to explain things to children: '*I mean usually ... you rely on the nurses a lot ... and ... we've got very good nurses and they are very friendly with the children and I think a lot of very young children find women more calming and less threatening than men anyway ... I think they [nurses] have a huge part to play; they're probably more effective than me in making the kid feel comfortable*' (HPII 15).

The problem of the lack of specialist training in children's healthcare for those dealing with children was a problem explained also by a nurse manager in a general hospital, who said: '*There are a lot of areas where nurses aren't paediatrically trained, there are doctors who aren't paediatric trained and we've no paediatric surgeon*' (HPGI 1). The consequence of this, she explained, is that '*teams of orthopaedic, neuro- or general surgeons are not children-oriented and thus children with these problems will be looked after by a consultant who mainly looks after adults. This means that the medical care of a significant number of children will be looked after by those who are not specifically trained in children's health*'. She described the significance of this as follows: '*Communication and child development, that's not their area, that's not their basic training. The child will be very well looked after if they need plastic surgery or need surgery. But communicating with the parent, communicating with the child will be lacking because they deal with adults mainly*' (HPGI 1).

Although progress had been made insofar as training in children's healthcare is required by everyone working within children's units, this contrasts clearly with the situation elsewhere, such as in England where '*you have to have paediatric nurses within every area*' (HPGI 1). This was important, as a nurse manager explained: '*There should be a paediatric nurse in X-ray. There should be a paediatric nurse in out-patients. I worked in the UK [where] ... you had to have a paediatric nurse within every area. And whereas here, when I came back, I couldn't believe it — there was no paediatric nurse and there was no paediatric-trained nurse in out-patients or in A&E*' (HPGI 1).

Willingness to undergo training

Many professionals expressed a willingness and interest in undertaking training on communicating with children. While maybe not entirely typical, a paediatric oncologist who is involved in education expressed his view as follows: '*I have no difficulty listening to any other experienced individual talking about this subject and indicating their methodology and outlining their own experience. I read widely on the subject and ... I don't think you can ever get to the point where you claim you know everything. And a lot of the time when you're communicating with this age group, regardless of how experienced you are, you're flying by the seat of your pants anyway. I mean, do any of us really know what people want to hear when they ask a question?*' (HPII 23).

Others, while willing to undergo training, questioned whether they would have the time. As one consultant dermatologist in this category explained: *'If I had time ... A lot of these things depend on what time you've got available in your working day. So if I had time, certainly'* (HPII 4). Others felt that they would only attend training that was of a particularly high standard. As one anaesthetist said: *'If the quality of the training was such that it merited inclusion, I would be delighted because I think it is a deficiency. But ... it could not be ad hoc or ... well intentioned. If it was a high quality training, yes'* (HPII 16).

Summary

The fact that many of the issues raised in this chapter have been identified already by either children or parents shows a consistency in the research carried out and the shared experiences and perspectives of all parties involved in children's health. The influential role of factors such as the personality and attitude of the health professional, the lack of training in communication skills and limited resources such as time and physical environment — all these are themes that resonate throughout the research. These must be addressed before children will be listened to by their health professionals.

The difference between the approaches of some health professionals — particularly those with specialist training in children's healthcare and those who have specialised in other areas but nonetheless treat children — is also clear. In addition to the need to address the training of all health professionals in this context, this also raises the need to adopt a common and multidisciplinary approach to communicating with children throughout the healthcare system. The different demands and challenges faced by health professionals must, however, be taken into account since all have different roles within the system, as well as different time and resources at their disposal.

Although the duty to listen to children is clearly placed on the shoulders of the health professional, this discussion confirms that the role of parents in the process is as influential in practice as in theory. Indeed, interviews with health professionals confirm that the dynamic between them and parents is a hugely significant factor in how they communicate with their child patients. The fact that, for many health professionals, parents' influence on the effectiveness of communication with children is decisive in both positive and negative terms means that any training of health professionals on listening to children must also address these tensions and how to deal with them.

8 EDUCATION AND TRAINING OF HEALTH PROFESSIONALS

In addition to recording the perspectives and experiences of children, parents and health professionals on listening to children in the healthcare sector, this research also sought to examine the education and training of health professionals in this area. This was undertaken in two ways:

- First, the core curricula of a number of educational courses were examined. Although the focus was primarily on medical training, the curricula of dentists, nurses, play specialists, speech and language therapists, and occupational therapists were also examined.
- Second, this analysis was supplemented by the data gathered during interviews with health professionals, including those involved in education and training, where they shared their experiences and views on the issue. In particular, the interviews sought to discover what training health professionals had received on communicating with children, to gauge the attitudes of professionals towards the clinical model of medical training and to measure their awareness of best practice or other guidelines from their profession on communicating with children.

This combined approach was important given that detailed information on the formal content of courses relevant to communicating with children was not always available. Moreover, information on the approaches of those involved in the teaching of communication skills to medical and healthcare students was provided during a round-table discussion dedicated to the topic at one of Ireland's medical schools.

The following discussion provides a useful barometer of the progress made in including communication skills on the curricula of a number of health professions, which is crucial if communication with children is to be included also.

As in Chapter 7, the same system is used here to identify the interview type and number during which the health professionals made their comments *(set in italics)*, i.e. HPGI (for Health Professionals Group Interview) and HPII (for Health Professional Individual Interview).

Experiences and attitudes of health professionals

During the course of this research, health professionals were interviewed about the level of training they had received on communicating with children and their attitudes to further training. The attitudes, training and experiences varied from profession to profession and so care is taken not to draw common conclusions across the entire healthcare setting. As a professor of speech therapy explained, the demands and approaches of medical professionals vary from one to another: *'We teach students how to develop a kind of therapeutic relationship that allows the client to let down some of those barriers. Of course, it's different to a doctor ... in a medical consultation who maybe has only 15 minutes to elicit information and the information is very specific ... to when you have to possibly spend up to an hour, or an hour and a half, making an assessment of a child's language disorder. So there are different constraints on different professions in terms of communication'* (HPGI 3).

With this diversity in mind, the following section details the views of health professionals on the significance of learning by experience, their lack of formal training and the current lack of resources in the area.

Professionals' experience of training and awareness of best practice guidelines

Most health professionals expressed the view that experience, rather than academic coursework, had taught them the necessary skills and techniques for communicating with children. Thus, many of the professionals reported that they had either received no communications training at all or none specific to children. Several professionals commented on the absence of training modules or professional guidelines in the area of communication with children. For example, one GP commented: *'In paediatrics, we would have done no specific module on communicating with children and I did the diploma in child health and to the best of my knowledge when I did it, which is now 12, 13 years ago, there was no module on communication skills'* (HPII 2).

Again, an anaesthetist said there was *'no specific training ... I never attended a course as to how to speak with children, speak to parents, speak to both beforehand, only insofar as that you work through the paediatric training that was part of our whole anaesthetic training'* (HPII 21).

Few health professionals expressed any awareness of particular models of communication and virtually none had had any formal training. A sample of views follows. One dermatologist said: *'I don't have a set way of doing it. I think you asked whether I had any training on this and I would say I haven't. It's purely from my own dealing with children in out-patients'* (HPII 4). A radiographer said: *'I was never trained on best practice or anything like that. Mine would be coming from experience'* (HPII 18). A play specialist said: *'I haven't actually been made aware of any particular models ... I suppose it's sort of what we were taught in college and just from experience you know'* (HPII 9).

These views were reiterated both by those who had done their training in the recent past and by those currently delivering education or training to students. An anaesthetist involved in education said: *'We don't offer formal training in communication with kids and that may well be a deficiency. But, like much of medical training, I think that would fall into the category of "one learns by observing experienced clinicians in action" '* (HPII 16). Similarly, a lecturer at a dental school explained the training that current dental students undertake: *'They spend the whole day basically learning communication skills on very much a hands-on basis, and we're with them every step of the way. We don't really have a formal section that deals with communication as such, even though I have been looking at it. We do have a seminar on it scheduled ... It's the first time it's being specifically taught, but we teach by example and ... by hands-on method really'* (HPII 3).

Many of the professionals interviewed reported that they had received formal training on communicating generally, but nothing specific to children. As a researcher nurse told us: *'In our training, we would have done ... communication skills, but not anything specific on communicating with children'* (HPII 13).

An ENT surgeon said that he did not receive any formal training in relation to communicating with children. On awareness of best practice in this context, he said: *'I haven't seen anything written down and I haven't been involved in any courses or anything like that ... I finished my training ... 12 years ago and we certainly didn't have anything like that'* (HPII 12). One GP commented that there were *'no guidelines in terms of communicating and consulting'* (HPII 2).

An anaesthetist said he was not really aware of best practice and felt that his own experience was the best guide: *'I suppose I trust my own common sense and experience really. I've been at it a long time now ... I think it's one of those things; if you've been at it a long time, I think you just naturally, by trial and error, eventually come to a technique that seems not to alarm people too much and works most of the time'* (HPII 15).

Another anaesthetist questioned whether guidelines or best practice for communication with children actually exist. He commented: *'What does exist is an entire litany of suggestions, recommendations at all sorts of levels from text books to experienced clinicians ... you know there's a certain amount of original research on the mode of communication with kids during the pre-operative period ... The research studies would be few and far between ... every paediatric and anaesthetic text will have a chapter or a section devoted to that'* (HPII 16).

A psychologist also referred to some academic education, but was less specific about its content or usefulness: *'I can't remember any academic content particularly about communicating with them [children], although I know there were some things ... that would have been specifically touched on when we were on our training'* (HPII 3).

It is clear from these reports, therefore, that communication with children is not a core part of the curriculum taught to health professionals, either in the past or present. Nor does it appear to form a core part of paediatric training. An important factor here is the prominence of the clinical model of education, where interns and other trainees learn on-the-job.

The clinical model of education

Many professionals expressed the view that medical education and training, particularly relating to communication and bedside manner, is something that is best learned on-the-job. For example, an A&E doctor said: *'I suppose, as an undergraduate in medical school ... we all get lectures in paediatrics and ... about six weeks' clinical attachment on the ward, where you actually met children.*

You worked with the team and you worked with the other doctors on the team. So they basically taught you. You got informal teaching and bedside teaching there, so that's where you got used to children' (HPII 6).

The view that communication skills were best learned during clinical training was widespread. A common view, expressed by a researcher nurse, was that good communication skills were inherent; they were then further developed or improved through practice (HPII 13). A lecturer in a dental school expressed a similar view: *'For some people it comes to them naturally — it's like riding a bicycle, once you know how to do it. But if you had to stop and explain, well, you put your foot here, it isn't easy to explain to somebody because you either have it or you haven't'* (HPGI 3).

However, not all professionals felt that the clinical model taught them everything they needed to know. One GP told us: *'The only model we have is when we do our paediatric training in hospitals. You follow the consultants and that isn't necessarily always a positive model'* (HPII 2).

This view was also expressed by the interns interviewed, who explained that seeing both bad practice as well as good practice had an impact on them. In relation to bad practice, one intern explained: *'It makes me more conscious. I'd think, Oh God! I'd never want to do that'* (HPII 2). Similarly, another intern identified that witnessing both good and bad practice among consultants was a learning experience, saying she had experienced both sides: *'Sometimes you're in situations and you go, Oh God! The way they handled that, and then other times, you'd say, Now, that was good! I'd like to think I'd be able to do it that way'* (HPII 2).

While it was useful to see bad practice that should not be emulated, the interns felt that they learned more from seeing best practice in operation. As one intern explained: *'It's probably easier ... to see somebody who does it well, maybe you do learn a bit more ... because you can pick up things from that. Whereas somebody who does it badly, you just know you don't want to do that, but you might not pick up the instruction'* (HPII 2).

The value of clinical-based education, in highlighting both good and bad practice, is clear from these experiences. While the clinical model of medical training has received attention in recent years, the need to incorporate communication skills formally into healthcare curricula is also gaining recognition *(see below)*. As well as the attitudes of health professionals to such an approach, as seen above, barriers to teaching communication skills are also relevant here.

Barriers to teaching communication skills

Barriers to teaching communication skills appear, from this research, to be varied. Factors such as a squeezed curriculum, a lack of appreciation for the importance of training in communication skills and a strong perception that such skills are innate rather than acquired — all these factors mitigate against the inclusion of communication skills in the medical curriculum.

Conversations with those involved in the provision of education to medical and other healthcare students clearly identified the limited time available as a barrier to the introduction into the curriculum of communication skills, including those with children (HPGI 3). For example, the pressure of completing the medical curriculum means that time for communication, rather than other medicine-related skills, is limited. This appeared to be a problem throughout all professions within the healthcare setting.

The lack of importance attached to communication skills was also identified as a problem in raising its profile or justifying its inclusion in undergraduate or continuing medical or healthcare education. For example, the difficulty for those seeking leave to undertake training was explained in one group discussion. As one lecturer explained: *'In a hospital that is understaffed ... the person who is leaving to get the training is perceived to be the enemy as opposed to the system being the enemy. And it's very short-sighted, but it happens'* (HPGI 3).

Children's nurses, who have received training on communicating with children, also questioned whether they were rated as highly as other nurse specialists. One children's nurse who had been trained in the UK explained: *'Well, I've only been here 18 months, but I found when I came back*

*that ... paediatrics wasn't held [in] as high esteem as midwifery ... But actually paediatrics ...
is as long a course and it's a diploma ... only obviously a different speciality'* (HPGI 1).

It was noted above that some health professionals perceive basic communication skills to be
innate rather than acquired. This was also acknowledged by those involved in the provision of
education to be the view of some students as well. As one lecturer in a nursing school explained:
*'The content [of the communications course] was seen as common sense ... We all think we have a
certain level of communication skills ... you're meant to have the skills already and I think students
have that kind of perception too'* (HPGI 3).

Some of those teaching communication skills to medical students shared this view. A lecturer at a
dental school explained: *'I just find some students are extremely poor at communicating and this is
one of the most difficult things to teach them, to actually teach them how to stand and talk to
somebody'* (HPGI 3).

While this comment was made with regard to general communication skills rather than
communication with children, it clearly applies to both situations. Course content is vital in this
context and this is acknowledged by those involved in medical education. According to some
educators, the ideal approach is to build on the skills that students already have, by focusing on
their awareness of their skills and developing related areas of expressing feelings of emotion and
empathy (HPGI 3).

Nonetheless, integrating communication skills into the curriculum is not easy and developing and
imposing formal assessment has been problematic too. As one professor of education involved in
GP education explained: *'It's a very controversial thing and it's deeply personal, so it's very difficult
to sit back in judgement and say "You're not a good communicator" or indeed "You're an inadequate
communicator". So ... we have to be very careful ... how far we go with that'* (HPGI 3).

At the same time, discussions among those involved in healthcare education explained the need
to use the theoretical models in existence and in use elsewhere to formally assess communication
skills in order to attribute them importance alongside other clinical and medical skills. It is clear,
therefore, that there is scope for the health professions to learn from each other in this area.

Linguistic and cultural issues
An important issue raised by one psychologist was the fact that increasing multiculturalism in Ireland
has highlighted linguistic and cultural issues relevant to effective communication with children. Her
view was that these issues have not been addressed by any education or training. She noted with
concern the 'cultural gap' that existed in one children's hospital and described the problem as
follows: *'We're dealing with so many people through so many languages or children [for] whom English
wouldn't be their first language, but also whose customs and suspicions of us would be so much higher
than an Irish child ... There'd [also] be our own different cultures, you know, the Travellers and ...
all the different things you'd get even within Ireland'* (HPII 3).

Further research is required to explore the challenges involved in delivering healthcare to a
multicultural population. Issues raised by Traveller parents in Chapter 6, however, highlight that
the link between cultural diversity and poor communication is not a new problem. While these
issues were addressed in the 2002 Traveller National Health Strategy, nonetheless, the experiences
of both parents and health professionals reported in this research support giving further
consideration to integrating training into the curriculum in this area.

Staff initiatives
In some specialities, there seemed to be a stronger emphasis on continuing education and
training, and an encouragement and facilitation of staff undertaking specialist training courses,
either on their own initiative or as part of their employment. For example, in the area of social
work, one practitioner working in paediatrics noted: *'There were skills labs on effective
communication and on child-centred communication. Limited, I would have to say. The more I've
come into paediatric social work ... I myself have undergone training around communication and*

*advocacy for children and understanding children's emotional responses to long-term illnesses ...
I suppose that's thanks to the Health Board's training and my own initiative. That wouldn't have
been part of the course ... I think it's an area that would warrant almost a specialist module a term
and it isn't there'* (HPII 1).

Another social worker reported the training she had undertaken, saying: *'During the initial training,
[we] would have lectures in developmental psychology and child psychology and ... during practice
[we] developed skills. Staff in recent years have undertaken some training in creative art therapy
when working with children'* (HPII 10).

In relation to how such training should best be given, a social worker recommended an integrated
approach, where communication with children would build on child psychology. She commented:
*'It's not something you learn in a little module ... you're going to have to have a good basis in child
psychology, for example, if you're going [to work with children] and this will be an add-on to that. But
you need to have a good base ... of understanding children's development, of understanding ... how
children operate and then communicating with children in a medical setting'* (HPII 10). In her view,
then, communicating with children needed to be integrated and mainstreamed throughout the
curriculum: *'It needs to be part of something that runs through, hopefully, all the training'* (HPII 10).

Medical education

There are five undergraduate medical schools in Ireland, based in University College Cork, National
University of Ireland Galway, Trinity College Dublin, University College Dublin, and the Royal
College of Surgeons. The medical schools have moved, or are currently moving, to 5-year degree
courses, which produce medical graduates who are conferred with degrees of MB (Bachelor of
Medicine), BCh (Bachelor in Surgery) and BAO (Bachelor in the Art of Obstetrics). On graduation,
the newly qualified doctor works as an intern in a recognised hospital, either in Ireland or
elsewhere. On completion of the internship, a Certificate of Experience is granted by the Dean of
the Medical School and the doctor is then entitled to full registration with the Medical Council of
Ireland. The doctor then goes on to spend several years training in a hospital or in the community
to become an independent specialist.

The Medical Council is obliged, under the terms of the Medical Practitioners Act, 1978, to satisfy
itself as to the content and delivery of medical education in Ireland. Part of this function involves
an evaluation and accreditation process, with school visits by teams comprised of medical and lay
persons, as well as Council members. Suggestions as to curriculum change are then made and
implemented by the schools. So, for example, the Council suggested in 2001 that changes be made
to incorporate the behavioural sciences and medical ethics into the curriculum. Most of these
suggestions have now been at least partially implemented in the medical schools (Medical Council
of Ireland, 2001).

The Council is of the view that medical education is best provided in small teaching groups, which
facilitate student interaction and help to develop interpersonal skills. However, the Council has
reported that, in some schools, reflection on curricula is weak and there are too many standalone
modules that are not integrated into the mainstream medical education. There is overemphasis on
medicine and surgery in the curricula and, although medical ethics has been incorporated into
most schools, it is often not integrated into clinical disciplines and does not allow for small group
interaction. There are also serious concerns that the behavioural sciences are not taught in an
integrated and sustained manner in the undergraduate courses (Medical Council of Ireland, 2004a).

It is clear that medical education in Ireland is currently in a state of flux. Concern has been
expressed regarding the serious underfunding of medical schools and the inflexibility of educational
structures that hinder the progress of curriculum change. Some schools recognise the necessity for
structural and curriculum change, and it is expected that this will continue to evolve and develop
over the next few years (Department of Health and Children, and Department of Education and
Science, 2006).

Teaching communication skills

Among the five medical schools, there is little evidence that communication strategies for children are taught at undergraduate level. There are modules on ethics, paediatrics and communication skills, all of which provide some information on the importance of listening to children and engaging them in their own healthcare. However, it appears that most doctors are expected to learn such skills through the apprenticeship model or on-the-job training.

Most texts on doctor-patient communication do not address communicating with children and adolescents, either in situations where a parent is also present or where the doctor is seeing an unaccompanied adolescent. Until recently, research into communication in paediatric settings has focused almost exclusively on parent-doctor communication, although some studies have explored the level of children's contributions and interaction during consultations with GPs and hospital consultants.

Clinical education

Communication skills appear to be taught through the approach of clinical education or on-the-job training. While this approach has clear advantages and disadvantages *(see below)*, it was clear from interviews with health professionals that those who themselves learned through the apprenticeship model are likely to see the advantages of learning from senior colleagues as supplementary to academic learning. For example, one Senior House Officer tutor was of the opinion that *'it's not something that can be learned from books, one is born with communication ability. Some of it is common sense, like getting down to the child's level — students learn this from their superiors'* (HPGI 3).

Interns explained how they acquire most skills during their clinical training, which was described as *'an ongoing kind of process where you just pick up ... from other people'* (HPGI 2). However, despite the effective and appropriate nature of clinical education, much depends on the team leader or consultant under whom an intern studies. For example, it was clear from the interviews with health professionals at all stages of their careers that not all had had good role models during their clinical education. Thus, while some learned how to enhance their communication skills during this time, others who undertook an internship under a consultant who did not consider good communication skills important were likely to see a decline in existing ability to communicate.

One health professional involved in education explained that an intern will normally be guided by the priority attached by the surgeon or anaesthetist, who may not be terribly interested in *'whether you found out about this person as a person, if you empathised with them or anything like that'*, but who will be more concerned if the intern has not found out the patient's blood pressure (HPGI 3). Similarly, interns recognised that lengthy experience did not necessarily equate with best practice: *'Sometimes I think it's lethargy. Maybe somebody has been there for a very long time and ... it's not necessarily a consultant or a registrar ... just different people ... it's like a kind of lethargy; they've been doing it so long, they think they are getting better'* (HPGI 2).

This is consistent with the evidence, which shows that rather than improve with time, communication skills may, in fact, worsen through exposure to poor role models, among other things. As one professor of education at a medical school explained: *'There are a number of studies looking at communication skills, medical students and doctors at different stages of their career and ... the study I know of ... showed [that] people coming into medical school often had quite good communication skills, [which] ... tend to deteriorate a little bit as they go through ... They collapse completely at the intern year and they gradually improve as they get on to the consultation bit, and get back on to the level they were at when they left school'* (HPGI 3).

Despite this, in general in medical schools, communication strategies are not dealt with in a focused or isolated manner. Students encounter the subject in an embedded way by undertaking focus workshops or seminars dealing with specific issues, such as history-taking or how to impart bad news. While the embedded nature of the subject makes it difficult to evaluate the extent of training medical students receive on communication skills, it may also mean that its importance is not highlighted sufficiently. As one professor involved in the training of GPs put it: *'The emphasis is substantially on the clinical, even though the communication [skills] are being assessed at the same time, and maybe that needs to be made a bit more explicit. And it may be that ... we could do more of this assessment as they go along and as they develop the skills'* (HPGI 3).

The understanding of the amount of communication skills taught may also be a case of what the education is called rather than its content (HPGI 3). However, it is clear that no differentiation appears to be made between adults and children in this context and that the relatively recent focus on communication skills does not, in all professions, include communicating with children. By comparison, modules on paediatrics tend to be described as small-group, patient-centred teaching, where students learn the skills of listening and communicating, history-taking and clinical examination. In one medical school, the objectives of the module on paediatrics include the development of the paediatric content of medical undergraduate curriculum to ensure that all medical graduates are sensitive to the needs of sick children. Interns interviewed for this research also described lectures they had received on child development and on how children express themselves (HPGI 2), although these lectures appeared to be ad hoc events rather than part of the curriculum.

Interns interviewed also attached value to combining theoretical with clinical education in this area. As one explained, the preferable approach was not to put everything down to experience, but to have a theoretical base on which to fall back: *'First, the theoretical, where you're told this and then, when you are on the floor as an intern, as a practitioner, then ... you put those kind of things into practice. Through the years, I think we would then pick up and develop our own sense of when to tell, how much not to tell ... So I know a lot of time they were saying that [for] the most senior staff it has to do with that experience and someday we will have that as well, but ... it is good that, starting off in med school, they actually address the issues'* (HPGI 2).

GP training
For many children, the only point of contact they may have during childhood and early adolescence is with their general practitioner (GP) or family doctor. All GPs follow the same basic training in medical school, before continuing on with further specialised vocational training for general practice, which would include modules on paediatrics and psychiatry.

A GP involved in the education of medical students in one medical school explained that *'medical students get 6 hours' communication skills throughout 5 years of medical school'* as part of an Anatomy module, although this represents only the formal, rather than the informal, training provided (HPGI 3). However, this training focuses on communication with adults as opposed to children, as the lecturer explained: *'Basically what we do is get them to role-play mock consultations, so we ask the students to pretend to be a doctor and we also ask them to pretend to be patients. We played a lot with the idea of having sort of formal role-plays for them, but in fact the stuff they actually come up with themselves is very innovative and I think they get a lot out of pretending to be a patient relating to some illness experience they might have had themselves ... And then we get the students to feedback to each other ... what's good about what they did, what they felt was good or could have been better, with feedback and comments from the group'* (HPGI 3).

Those interviewed acknowledged that the time allowed for this training was limited, not least because every medical student did not get the opportunity to play the role of the health professional. As another GP involved in education explained: *'The overall time ... is only 6 hours, so we try within the 6 hours to make sure that every student is at least on camera in one or other role. Now, it would be preferable that each of them would get both roles and we have a longer time for discussion but ... what we don't pick up with one student, we pick up with another'* (HPGI 3).

Education on communication theory is also provided, but this too has limitations in the current educational framework. As a GP explained: *'We also participate in another module called behavioural science and that is actually where we talk a little bit about theory on communication. But again, that's fairly light; it sort of talks a little bit about verbal and non-verbal communication, that sort of thing. But again at a very basic level'* (HPGI 3).

In public health nursing, guidelines are set down at national and regional levels as to the role of the public health nurse and how to engage with children, normally through parental consent. As one public health nurse explained: *'You bring to public health nursing the academic and the experiential learning ... communication skills and the verbal and non-verbal cues, the listening. We would have the theory of it and you just put that into practice ... If everyone had a degree in psychology, it certainly would help, particularly the whole-child psychological development and communication skills'* (HPII 7).

Dentists

Dental training in Ireland involves a 5-year degree course, which combines academic study with clinical experience. Typically, students spend the first third of their time in academic study and the remaining time involves clinical training. Dental training courses are offered in Trinity College Dublin and University College Cork. Both these dental schools also offer dental nurse training.

From a review of the curricula of the dental schools, it would appear that, as with the training of doctors, the teaching of communication skills is through the apprenticeship model. It was described by one lecturer in a dental hospital as *'sadly lacking'* (HPII 22). This commentator recognised the disadvantages of not having any formal course in communication skills, but pointed to the lack of funding to introduce modules dealing with issues such as behavioural science (HPII 22). In the module descriptions for dentistry in one university, there are topics such as diagnostic assessment, obtaining history, legal requirements (insurance and malpractice issues) and ethics (behaviour and conduct issues), but there is no reference to communication or child patients.

The difficulties experienced by dentists in relation to communication with children are similar to those expressed by their medical colleagues in terms of information deficit, fear or vulnerability on the part of the child, parental reaction, lack of cooperation, time management and so on. In terms of guidelines or training in this context, one paediatric dentist told us: *'I'm not 100% sure about guidelines specifically for speaking with a child. We're examining the training programme at the moment and the way specialists are trained in paediatric dentistry. So we get advice from [the] management style of techniques for speaking with children and about treating them as well'* (HPII 22).

The same dentist described his experience as a student: *'What we had was this thing called behaviour management ... We get papers ... on how kids learn and how best to use the learning and coping skills at different ages and what you can actually do with different ages. Because we would also see the young kids as well as 4-year-olds'* (HPII 22). This dentist also described the topic of communicating with children as being the focus of conferences and lectures.

Nurses

Nurse education has been the subject of much debate over the last decade since concerns were raised regarding the appropriateness of the apprenticeship model for their education and training. A Commission on Nursing was established in 1997 to examine and report on the role and function of nurses and midwives in the context of anticipated changes in the organisation and delivery of the Irish health service.

In its *Blueprint for the Future* report, published in 1998, the Commission recommended that nurses be educated by way of a 4-year degree programme, which would provide both the theoretical and clinical competency required (Commission on Nursing, 1998). The Commission also suggested that theoretical work must not be less than one-third of the recommended course and clinical work not less than half. Furthermore, specialist placements within the clinical component must comprise not less than one-quarter of the clinical learning time, with at least 2 weeks in each component. These placements include Accident & Emergency, child care paediatrics, mental health, elderly care, home nursing, crèche facilities, theatre and maternity care.

Degree courses in nursing (BSc in Nursing Studies) are now offered by all the Irish universities (Trinity College Dublin; University College Dublin; University College Cork; University of Limerick; National University of Ireland Galway; and Dublin City University), as well as the Royal College of Surgeons and the Institute of Technology, Tralee. In 2006, a new integrated general and children's nursing programme will commence in University College Cork. Currently, specialist child nursing post-graduate courses are offered by University College Dublin (which offers a Higher Diploma in Sick Children's Nursing) and Trinity College Dublin (which offers a Post-graduate Diploma in Paediatric Nursing). Graduates of these programmes may be registered as Sick Children's Nurses (RSCN) with An Bord Altranais (the Irish Nursing Board).

Most BSc degree courses offer modules specifically targeted at communication, in which models of interpersonal communication are demonstrated and applied to specific patient situations. For example, in University College Cork, there are a number of modules offered on the BSc course which develop students' communication skills. These include modules on Interpersonal Communication (which has components on theoretical consideration; interpersonal and intrapersonal; relational, situational and cultural factors; skills in differing patient situations; self-awareness); Interpersonal Skills for Nursing Practice (which has components on human communication, including levels of communication; theories and models of interpersonal communication; factors influencing interpersonal communication; and application of interpersonal communication to specific patient/client situations); Therapeutic Interpersonal Skills and Social Psychology for Nursing (which includes components on nursing as a therapeutic-interpersonal process).

In addition to these modules, which appear to address communication issues across a range of patients, the modules relating specifically to children also indicate an awareness of the importance of communication and an acknowledgement of the rights of children. For example, the module on Maternity Care and Child Health Nursing includes components on the growing and developing child, on family-centred care and on the child as consumer and participant in healthcare.

A nurse, involved in delivery of nursing education at one of the universities, commented: *'There have been dedicated modules on interpersonal skills for nursing at least since the diploma came in in 1997, so we have been teaching it to nurses for at least that number of years, if not before that as well'* (HPGI 3).

Typically, the communications course involves a combination of lectures and small-group tutorials, using role-plays, interactive teaching and focusing on specific scenarios such as communicating with people with sensory disability. The specific challenge of communicating with children, however, does not appear to have dedicated time. In some courses, student nurses also now do a module on children's play needs.

Some children's nurses interviewed for this research referred to the theoretical foundation upon which their practices were built. One nurse said: *'There's an awful lot of theories in relation to communication ... I've a degree in cancer nursing and certainly we would have looked at communication skills and done assignments in relation to that and different theories and obviously understanding of a child through their different milestones and what they understand at various levels'* (HPII 20).

Specialised communication skills is also a subject in the post-graduate diplomas. In these diplomas, the social, psychological and theoretical aspects of communication are also emphasised. The curriculum for the Higher Diploma in Sick Children's Nursing, offered by University College Dublin, provides a useful example of the approach taken in this area. This 78-week Diploma is offered in conjunction with Our Lady's Hospital for Sick Children, Crumlin, and the Children's University Hospital, Temple Street. In addition to modules relating to the healthcare needs of children, the Diploma offers a range of modules to enhance the students' understanding of their patients' broader needs, both personally and within their family units.

In this regard, relevant modules taken include Child and Family Centred Nursing; Theoretical Foundations of Sick Children's Nursing; Child and Family Health Promotion; and Social and Behavioural Sciences. The last of these modules contains a specific component on communication skills, as well as covering the child and family in society; social policy and social administration; developmental psychology in infancy, childhood and adolescence; and the child with altered psychological and psychiatric function. Furthermore, as part of a module on Professional and Contemporary Issues in Child Health, students take components on the legal and ethical aspects of sick children's nursing, as well as dealing with professional and management issues. It is clear that communication with and understanding of children and young people is made central in the holistic approach adopted by this kind of nursing course.

Training for other health professionals

Speech and Language Therapists

Degree courses for the speciality of speech and language therapy are run in Trinity College Dublin, University of Limerick and University College Cork. The second year is focused on paediatrics, with an emphasis on development and linguistic issues from a clinical and theoretical perspective. Students engage in role-play and video consultations to identify best practice and to develop and assess communicative abilities in those being trained. Education is problem-based, using clinical scenarios to trigger the issues to be focused upon. Training on communication skills, including with children and their parents, is embedded in clinical placement modules rather than taught as a separate module (HPGI 3). To this extent, the students' curriculum is entirely communication-based.

As a professor in the area explained: *'There are a number of analytical research tools that can also be used to analyse communications. For example, things like discourse analysis, conversation analysis are actually research methodologies used by researchers to analyse clinical interactions and that kind of thing. And also to analyse interactions of people with communication disorders and ordinary people without communication disorders. So those actual methods of analysing, looking at things like developing, having a taxonomy of communication acts like asking for information, delivering information, making a statement, making a promise — all these things can be analysed into their different components. And that's referred to as discourse analysis, communication, conversation analysis. So those kinds of things are taught in research methodology to our students on how to analyse interactions between people'* (HPGI 3).

The professor continued: *'One of the important things we do is also teach our students to analyse non-verbal communications, so we actually go into communication theory, looking at things like proximics, what is acceptable in social distances, how close you can sit to a client without causing offence and how different cultures interpret those proximics depending on whether it's social distance or intimate distance'* (HPGI 3).

Occupational Therapists

Degree courses for occupational therapy are offered in Trinity College Dublin, University of Limerick (post-graduate) and University College Cork (UCC). Occupational therapy trainees undertake communication skills training as an embedded part of their curriculum (HPGI 3). Significantly, in the second year of their studies at UCC, students focus specifically on children and young adults, and — in contrast to other health professionals whose educational curricula were examined for this research — on communication with children, including observing interactions between children and play, undertaking role-play with children and parents, and reflecting on how best to engage with children and their families (HPGI 3).

Courses follow a theoretical and a task-based teaching format, meeting people and interviewing and assessing children. The students provide feedback to instructors and reflect on their communication strategies with children. Parents are also involved in providing feedback on the experience to the students. Students also benefit from group work with speech and hearing sciences students, focusing on early child communication and how to communicate with young children and pre-schoolers.

Play Specialists

In Ireland, there are a number of play specialists who work with children in hospitals around the country. They receive specialist training in the East Antrim Institute. Their training in communicating with children includes both the theoretical framework and practical guidance, such as body language, tone and physical demeanour. One specialist commented on their approach: *'... using simple terminology, especially with medical areas, you explain procedures to them in the way that they will understand'* (HPII 9).

One play specialist commented that there should be more training and guidance available for all healthcare staff in terms of the differences between communicating with children and adults: *'It certainly would be more beneficial if there was more education made available to the different staff members who work with children in a healthcare setting … Some staff would not have very much experience with children because whatever job they do they cover all ages within the hospital. And I'm sure they would say as well that it's difficult … to make the switch if you're coming from an adult ward to a paediatric ward, then it's a completely different way of communicating'* (HPII 9).

Ethical standards and codes of conduct

In addition to the education and training curricula, some health professionals may also be guided by their codes of conduct and behaviour with regard to communication with children.

The Medical Council of Ireland's Guide to Ethical Conduct and Behaviour (2004b) provides the following guidelines to professionals. Under the heading 'Children', it states: 'If the doctor feels that a child will understand a proposed medical procedure, information or advice, this should be explained fully to the child. Where the consent of parents or guardians is normally required in respect of a child for whom they are responsible, due regard must be had to the wishes of the child. The doctor must never assume that it is safe to ignore the parental/guardian interest.'

The *Code of Conduct* of the Irish Nursing Board (1988) is a much less detailed document. No guidance is given in it regarding interaction with children.

In the UK, the Royal College of Paediatrics and Child Health has issued detailed guidance to its members, setting out the paediatrician's obligations in dealing with patients (RCPCH, 2002). In the section headed 'Relationship with patients', the guidelines state: 'You must respect the right of patients to be fully involved in decisions about their care. Wherever possible, you must be satisfied, before you provide treatment or investigate a patient's condition, that the patient has understood what is proposed, and why, and any significant risks or side-effects associated with it and has given consent.'

The guidelines are very clear that when a child is old enough to understand, they must be involved in discussions about their treatment. However, not all professionals interviewed in this research were aware of the existence and/or relevance of these RCPCH guidelines.

Increased importance of communication skills

It is clear that awareness of the importance of teaching communication skills at undergraduate level is increasing among those involved in the provision of education to the medical and health professions. Some interviewees recognised that the emphasis on communication skills has changed in recent times. As one clinical tutor put it: *'It's interesting that … when I was a medical student communication skills weren't taught at all … You were expected, because you were becoming a doctor, to have communication skills and over the years there has become a greater and greater interest in it'* (HPGI 3).

Today, there is a clear awareness of the importance of such skills. As one lecturer involved in teaching speech and language therapy students explained: *'If you think about it, when you go to your GP, for example, the thing that the patient experiences is communication … so … it's … an important aspect of the curriculum. I mean … knowing all that theory [is vital], but … the contact with the public is the thing'* (HPGI 3).

A nurse manager also explained how training has changed for nurses in recent times: *'For student nurses, there's … a paediatric module and they do a module on play. The student doctors rotate once in the playroom … They make it part of their training, so it is changing'* (HPGI 2).

Yet, for those training GPs, the focus on communication and its formal integration into the curriculum is still a new phenomenon. As one professor of education at a medical school explained, its inclusion in the curriculum does not mean that it is formally assessed or that equal weight is attached to it as to medical assessment: *'It certainly was the case, historically, that the first time their actual communications skills performance was assessed was at the very end of the course. It was far from ideal. But we are working on that and there are things happening'* (HPGI 3). He added that the teaching of communication skills, even involving adults, was at a developmental stage, but it is *'something that will get further developed as attention is given to this whole thing of communication skills as a sort of separate topic or a separate entity'* (HPGI 3).

Regarding the techniques used for teaching communication skills, new approaches are being piloted in some medical schools. For example, attempts are being made to introduce a patient perspective into medical training, whereby the patient group, called Patient Focus, has contributed to students' theoretical training. While more difficult to undertake in respect of children, this is certainly an approach worthy of replication throughout other medical schools and areas of training (HPGI 3).

The exchange of experiences and approaches among those involved in the various healthcare professions is particularly important in this context. It is especially relevant that those already engaged in teaching skills of communicating with children (including nursing, occupational, speech and language therapies) encourage interdisciplinarity with their colleagues involved in providing education to the medical professions.

The recognition of the importance of teaching communication skills as a formal part of the medical curriculum is clearly increasing and this is to be welcomed. However, the importance of also incorporating education on skills for communicating with children as a part of this approach does not appear to have gained widespread recognition. Nonetheless, there is considerable scope for developing curricula in this area at both undergraduate and post-graduate levels.

The UK experience

In the United Kingdom, following the publication of a report into cardiac surgery at the Bristol Royal Infirmary (2001), one of the key messages disseminated to health professionals was to involve children and families in healthcare decisions. It was recognised that new staff may get training in communication skills, but that existing staff may be anxious about their communication skills. Following from this public inquiry, some UK hospitals and NHS Trusts began to develop new strategies for education and training of professionals in this area.

For example, a pilot project was undertaken at Great Ormond Street Children's Hospital over a 3-month period to improve competence in communications. The project aimed to provide skills that would provide the tools for communication rather than focusing on one topic, such as delivering bad news. To achieve the objectives of the project, it was emphasised that the training should not be profession-specific, but should concentrate on generic skills, such as active listening, guiding an interview, avoiding premature reassurance and the provision of difficult information. It should also aim to engage members of multidisciplinary teams.

The objective of the NHS Trusts in relation to training strategies is to improve communication between clinicians and children and families. There is a demonstrable need for culture change in many hospitals following the reports in Bristol and in Alder Hey (Royal Liverpool Children's NHS Trust, 2004). Bereavement support is recognised as not being the only issue, and that good teamwork and communication is better for families and lessens the need for specialist referral. The catchwords here are 'Engagement', 'Reciprocity' and 'Partnership'. It is recognised that appropriate skills, consistently applied, make a difference to the quality of engagement between staff and families, leading to more patient-centred discussion, shared decision-making and greater confidence and clarity, in addition to greater patient satisfaction and compliance.

Summary

It is apparent from this discussion that no single conclusion can be drawn regarding the training of health professionals on communication with children. Indeed, this research shows that there is a notable difference between the education and training of nurses and therapists, on the one hand, and that of the medical and dentistry professions on the other. With regard to the latter, it must be acknowledged that clinical medical education, which is currently largely undocumented, may indeed incorporate the practice of communicating with children. Moreover, improvements and changes to curricula in the medical profession in particular are ongoing and may bring about further developments in this area in the near future.

With regard to the nursing profession and others, including occupational therapists and speech and language therapists, these professions appear to have made greater progress in the incorporation into their educational programmes of theoretical and practical approaches to listening to children. While at an early stage of development, best practice nonetheless appears to exist in the education and training of these professions, with the formal integration of communicating with children into their educational programmes.

In contrast, analysis of educational curricula for the medical profession indicates a lack of detailed or structured focus on either the theoretical or practical framework within which the voice of the child can effectively be heard in the healthcare setting. To date, the medical profession appears to have made more modest progress towards the incorporation of communication skills into education and training curricula, and has developed very limited, if any, training programmes on communicating with children.

Interviews with health professionals confirm the lacuna in their training in this regard, as well as the lack of guidance from their professional bodies on the topic, confirmed by the codes of conduct outlined above. Many health professionals who had not experienced any training on communicating with children had developed their own methodologies through emulation of senior colleagues, on-the-job training and reflection on specific case histories with clinical colleagues. Those who had experienced training took a more structured and perhaps formalised approach in their communication with children.

In light of the mixed progress towards incorporating communicating with children into the education and training curricula of health professionals, it is significant that awareness of the need for such training is on the increase. The current state of change of the medical curriculum in particular means that the time is opportune for cooperation within the healthcare setting in this area. While different approaches will be required in different areas, considerable good practice, which is equally relevant and appropriate to all professions, can be shared widely. The mainstreaming of theoretical and practical knowledge on how to communicate effectively with children is to be strongly encouraged.

In addition to developing competencies in this area, however, a broader issue arises with regard to the need to raise awareness of children's rights among all health professionals and the need to establish a common understanding of the importance and value of respecting the right of children to be heard. In this regard, training and education for health professionals must aim to develop both the skills to communicate effectively with children *and* the attitude and mind-set necessary to achieve greater respect for their rights in practice. The need to incorporate such training into the education of health professionals, as well as to integrate it into continuing professional development programmes, is evident from this research. Its clear relationship to the clinical skills, so important to all health professionals, may help to encourage already stretched practitioners of the importance of undertaking such training.

9 CONCLUSIONS AND RECOMMENDATIONS

The principal aim of this research was to evaluate, by means of qualitative research, the extent to which children's voices are being heard in the healthcare setting. It did this within a legal framework, which acknowledges that the child has a legal right to be heard and to have his or her views taken into account in all matters concerning him or her, but also within the perspective of medical law and issues of legal and general consent.

Following interviews with 51 children, 30 parents and 50 health professionals exploring experiences and attitudes in the area, the research undertook an audit of the education and teaching curricula of a range of health professionals. It also highlighted the views of those involved in this training, as well as the perspectives of other health professionals to the provision of training in this area.

Many conclusions were drawn throughout this report as to what needs to be done to implement the right of children to be heard in the healthcare setting. This discussion aims to reiterate briefly the positive initiatives identified by all groups interviewed regarding approaches to communicating effectively with children and the obstacles or barriers that exist to mainstreaming this best practice. It also draws conclusions on the education and training of health professionals and, in the final section, makes recommendations regarding ways of enhancing the profile of children in the healthcare setting and ensuring their voice is heard in line with Article 12 of the UN Convention on the Rights of the Child and the National Children's Strategy.

Findings

Views of children

The children interviewed for this research varied in age, gender, background and the level of contact they had had with the healthcare system. Yet, despite these variables, they consistently identified the importance of being heard by health professionals and routinely explained the importance to them of being provided with age-appropriate explanations and information to help them cope with the consultation and treatment process. They consistently articulated a need to be understood and, overwhelmingly, to be treated with empathy, kindness and good humour during illness, whether serious or not so serious. The children interviewed identified a range of reasons, both practical and principled, regarding why this was the case.

Interviews with children showed a variation in the extent to which their preferred model of participation matched the reality of their experience. While more extensive research is required before definitive conclusions can be reached, it appears from this research at least that children who have come into contact with specialists in children's health or those working in children's hospitals had more favourable experiences in this regard, in that they were better informed and more involved in their healthcare decisions.

Children also made valuable suggestions on how their interactions with health professionals could be improved. While many of the children referred specifically to their doctor in this regard, their recommendations — to undertake training with regard to effective communication with children and to use age-appropriate language and props — were directed at all health professionals, including nurses and dentists. Children's other recommendations — that waiting areas and hospitals be made more child-friendly, particularly for older children — are simple, yet clearly worthy of attention. All of these findings are consistent with research carried out elsewhere.

Views of parents

A diverse group of parents were interviewed, including some who were parents of the children interviewed and others who were unrelated. Their views on their experiences of attending health professionals with their children were rich and varied. It is perhaps simplistic to conclude that the views of those with a high level of contact with the healthcare system (such as those whose children have long-term and serious health problems) show a greater awareness of the importance of their child's participation in the consultation and treatment processes. However, on the basis of interviews with parents, greater involvement with the health professional does seem to impact on parental views on participation, together with other factors such as the fact that a child undergoing long-term treatment will develop and mature throughout this process.

More generally, a range of factors clearly affect the parents' views of the child's capacity and readiness to be fully involved in any communication with health professionals, not least the parents' own understanding of the process and of the right of their child to participate in it. An important issue identified in the interviews is the conflict that can arise between the parent and the health professional about the process of consulting and informing the child about their health and healthcare. This has been identified in other research of this kind. This research found that parents who did not appreciate health professionals' attempts to involve their child directly in the process were motivated by a variety of reasons, including a lack of awareness of the child's need and right to be involved and the need to protect the child from unnecessary anxiety. This demonstrates the complexity of the issue. It also highlights the importance of raising awareness among parents about the child's right to be heard and the need to ensure that health professionals receive the necessary skills and training on how to communicate with both parents and children in this setting.

At the same time, parents' identification of the need to adapt the hospital environment for children is entirely consistent with children's own views, as is their recommendation that health professionals need to show greater empathy with their child patients, to build relations with them based on trust and to communicate more directly with them. The need to provide training for health professionals in this area is also entirely consistent with the recommendation of children and the health professionals themselves. This is one area where unanimity was found to exist between all parties interviewed.

Views of health professionals

Many of the issues raised by health professionals were already identified in the interviews with children or parents, showing a consistency in the research carried out and the shared experiences and perspectives of all parties involved in children's health. The influential role of factors such as the personality and attitude of the health professional, the lack of training in communication skills and limited resources, such as time and physical environment, are all themes that resonate throughout the research. These obvious barriers to participation have also been clearly identified in other similar research.

Another finding of this research was the clear difference that exists between the approaches of some professionals, particularly those with specialist training in children's healthcare and those who have specialised in other areas, but nonetheless treat children. In addition to the need to address the training of all health professionals in this context, this also raises the need to adopt a common and multidisciplinary approach to communicating with children throughout the healthcare system. The different demands and challenges faced by health professionals must, however, be taken into account since all have different roles within the system, as well as different time and resources at their disposal.

Although the duty to listen to children is clearly placed on the shoulders of the health professional, interviews with the professionals themselves confirm that the role of parents in the process is as influential in practice as in theory. Indeed, consistent with other research, interviews with health professionals confirm that the dynamic between them and parents is a hugely significant factor in how they communicate with their child patients. The fact that, for many health professionals, parents' influence on the effectiveness of communication with children is decisive in either positive or negative terms means that any training of health professionals on listening to children must also address these tensions and how to deal with them.

Education and curriculum review

No single conclusion can be drawn about the extent to which the training of health professionals on communication with children meets the demands of Article 12 of the UN Convention on the Rights of the Child. According to this research, there is a notable difference between the education and training of nurses and therapists, on the one hand, and that of the medical and dentistry professions on the other. With regard to the latter, it must be acknowledged that clinical medical education, which is currently largely undocumented, may indeed incorporate the practice of communicating with children, but the lack of documentation made it difficult to measure. Moreover, improvements and changes to curricula in the medical profession in particular are ongoing and may bring about further developments in this area in the near future.

With regard to the nursing profession and others, including occupational therapists and speech and language therapists, these professions appear to have made greater progress in the incorporation into their educational programmes of theoretical and practical approaches to listening to children. While at an early stage of development, best practice nonetheless appears to exist in the education and training of these professions, with the formal integration of communicating with children into their educational programmes. In contrast, analysis of educational curricula for the medical profession indicates a lack of detailed or structured focus on either the theoretical or practical framework within which the voice of the child can effectively be heard in the healthcare setting. To date, the medical profession appears to have made more modest progress towards the incorporation of communication skills into education and training curricula, and has developed very limited, if any, training programmes on communicating with children.

Interviews with health professionals confirm the lacuna in their training in this regard, as well as the lack of guidance from their professional bodies on the topic, confirmed by the codes of conduct outlined in Chapter 8. Many health professionals who had not experienced any training on communicating with children had developed their own methodologies through emulation of senior colleagues, on-the-job training and reflection on specific case histories with clinical colleagues. Those who had experienced training took a more structured and perhaps formalised approach in their communication with children.

In light of the mixed progress towards incorporating communicating with children into education and training curricula of health professionals, it is significant that awareness of the need for such training is on the increase. The current state of change of the medical curriculum in particular means that the time is opportune for cooperation within the healthcare setting in this area. While different approaches will be required in different areas, considerable good practice, which is equally relevant and appropriate to all professions, can be shared widely. The mainstreaming of theoretical and practical knowledge on how to communicate effectively with children is to be strongly encouraged.

In addition to developing competencies in this area, however, a broader issue arises with regard to the need to raise awareness of children's rights among all health professionals and the need to establish a common understanding of the importance and value of respecting the right of children to be heard. In this regard, training and education for health professionals must aim to develop both the skills to communicate effectively with children *and* the attitude and mind-set necessary to achieve greater respect for their rights in practice. The need to incorporate such training into the education of health professionals, as well as to integrate it into continuing professional development programmes, is evident from this research. Its clear relationship to the clinical skills, so important to all health professionals, may help to encourage already stretched practitioners of the importance of undertaking such training.

Best practice in communicating with children

Chapter 1 set out the parameters of best practice against which the experiences of children, parents and health professionals were measured in the rest of this report. It is useful to reiterate the summary of best practice on communicating with children:

- The child must be involved in treatment decisions as far as possible, bearing in mind his or her capacity to understand and willingness to be involved.
- The patient's parents or carers must be involved in treatment decisions.
- The views of children must be sought and taken into account.
- The relationship between healthcare professional and child should be based on truthfulness, clarity and awareness of the child's age and maturity.
- Children must be listened to and their questions responded to, clearly and truthfully.
- Communication with children must be an ongoing process.
- Training in communication skills with children is an essential component of appropriate professional education.

In this research, children, parents and health professionals identified a wide range of approaches for listening to children in the healthcare setting. Regardless of their different perspectives, there was a remarkable degree of consistency between the models favourably identified in this context and the best practice identified above, although some parents were critical about professionals who, they believed, marginalised them from the process.

Best practice was found throughout the healthcare system among specialists in children's health and non-specialists, in both general and specialist children's hospitals. While positive initiatives were identified in all areas of the healthcare profession examined, positive experiences were more likely among those who had been trained in children's health and/or those who worked in a specialist environment (unit or hospital) for children.

The positive initiatives shown by health professionals can be summarised as follows:

- Addressing children directly during the consultation process (e.g. asking them personally about their ailment or condition). This is important regardless of the child's age, although the level of complexity, amount of information imparted and involvement of children in any decision-making process should be appropriate to the child's age and maturity. Although this will depend on the setting, efforts to communicate directly with children should not exclude parents and vice versa.
- Adopting an age-appropriate approach to treating children, which takes into account their development and capacity to understand.
- Chatting with the child to make them feel relaxed, while also respecting personal boundaries.
- Preparing children adequately for what is about to happen in a treatment or procedure, and giving them the opportunity to ask questions and to prepare themselves.
- Empathising with children, being light-hearted and good-humoured where appropriate.
- Using age-appropriate language and props to explain things to children, including their condition, the prescribed treatment or the procedure about to be undertaken.
- Giving children choices as to how they want to proceed.
- Being honest with children in order to build a relationship of trust.
- Creating an environment in which children are encouraged to ask questions.
- Making the healthcare environment, including waiting rooms and treatment areas, child-friendly for children of all ages.

Obstacles to communicating with children

Similar to the findings on the subject of best practice (see above), the research also identified, with remarkable consistency, what the obstacles are that currently prevent children being listened to in the healthcare setting. While some of these barriers are attitudinal and will require some time and effort to break down, others are structural and could be addressed with the appropriate use of resources. Some are within the gift of the health professionals themselves, while others fall under the responsibility of the Department of Health and Children. These barriers to communication include:

- **Training and experience:** While children's specialists appeared to be aware of and practise best practice regarding communicating with children, few non-specialists have received adequate training or education on children's rights, child development or ways of listening effectively to children in the healthcare setting. On-the-job training is not always an appropriate or effective way of providing this experience and has limitations that must be recognised in this context.
- **Intervention of parents:** The attitude and approach of parents can play both a negative and a positive role in the relationship between their child and the health professional, and can be decisive as to whether children are listened to in the healthcare setting.
- **Time:** The limited time available for consultations means that professionals do not have as long as they might need to ensure children are heard during the consultation and treatment process.
- **Physical environment:** The lack of available and appropriate space hinders effective communication between health professionals and their child-patients.
- **Personality of the health professional:** The personality or attitude of individual health professionals often plays a significant role as to whether or not they listen to children.

Recommendations

The following recommendations are made with a view to addressing the obstacles and challenges that currently exist to listening to children in the healthcare setting:

1. **Public information campaign:** A public information campaign aimed at children and adults needs to take place to raise awareness of the right of the child to be heard.

2. **Training:** Child development, children's rights and appropriate ways to communicate with children of all ages and stages of development should be incorporated into the training of all health professionals. This should also address the role of parents in this process.

3. **Protocols and best practice:** Protocols need to be developed between all health professionals, establishing best practice and shared approaches to communicating with children.

4. **Research:** Further research should be undertaken into the extent to which children are listened to in the healthcare setting. In particular, the experiences of teenagers and children and young people with disabilities should be taken into account.

BIBLIOGRAPHY

Alderson, P. (1993) *Children's Consent to Surgery.* Buckingham: Open University Press.

Alderson, P. and Montgomery, J. (1996) *Healthcare Choices: Making decisions with children.* London: Institute for Public Policy Research.

Angst, D.B. and Deatrick, J.A. (1996) 'Involvement in Healthcare Decisions: Parents and children with chronic illness', *Journal of Family Nursing,* Vol. 2, No. 2, pp. 174-94.

Backett, K. and Alexander, H. (1991) 'Talking to young children about health: Methods and findings', *Health Education Journal,* Vol. 50, No. 1, pp. 34-38.

Baker, H. (2005) 'Involving children and young people in research on domestic violence and housing', *Journal of Social Welfare and Family Law,* Vol. 28, Nos. 3-4, pp. 281-97.

Beauchamp, T. and Childress, J. (2001) *Principles of biomedical ethics* (6th edition). Oxford: Oxford University Press.

Beresford, B.A. and Sloper, P. (2003) 'Chronically ill adolescents' experiences of communicating with doctors: A qualitative study', *Journal of Adolescent Health,* Vol. 33, No. 3, pp. 172-79.

Brazier, M. and Bridge, C. (1996) 'Coercion or Caring: Analysing adolescent autonomy', *Legal Studies,* Vol. 16, p. 84.

Bricher, G. (1999) 'Children and Qualitative Research Methods: A review of the literature related to interview and interpretive processes', *Nurse Researcher,* Vol. 6, No. 4, pp. 65-77.

Bristol Royal Infirmary Inquiry (2001) *Learning from Bristol: The Report of the Public Inquiry into Children's Heart Surgery at the Bristol Royal Infirmary 1984-1995,* Command Paper: CM 5207. Bristol: Bristol Royal Infirmary Inquiry. Available at www.bristol-inquiry.org.uk

British Medical Association (2001) *Consent, rights and choices in health care for children and young people.* London: British Medical Association.

Broome, M.E. and Stieglitz, K.A. (1992) 'The Consent Process and Children', *Research in Nursing and Health,* Vol. 15, pp. 147-52.

Christensen, P. and James, A. (eds) (2000) *Research with Children: Perspectives and Practices.* London: Routledge Falmer.

Commission on Nursing (1998) *Report of the Commission on Nursing: A Blueprint for the Future.* Dublin: The Stationery Office. Available at www.dohc.ie

Committee on the Welfare of Children in Hospital (1959) *Report of the Committee.* London: HMSO.

Connolly, P. (2003) *Ethical Principles for Researching Vulnerable Groups.* Belfast: Office of the First Minister and Deputy First Minister of the Northern Ireland Assembly.

Cormack, J., Marinker, M. and Morrell, D. (eds) (1981) *Teaching General Practice.* London: Kluwer Medical.

Department of Health and Children (1999) *Children First: National Guidelines for the Protection and Welfare of Children.* Dublin: The Stationery Office.

Department of Health and Children (2000) *The National Children's Strategy: Our Children — Their Lives.* Dublin: The Stationery Office.

Department of Health and Children (2002) *Traveller Health: A National Strategy 2002-2005.* Dublin: The Stationery Office.

Department of Health and Children (2005) *Ireland's Second Report to the UN Committee on the Rights of the Child.* Dublin: The Stationery Office.

Department of Health and Children, and Department of Education and Science (2006) *Medical Education in Ireland: A New Direction. Report of the Working Group on Undergraduate Medical Education and Training,* chaired by Professor P. Fottrell. Dublin: The Stationery Office. Available at www.health.ie & www.education.ie

Donnelly, M. (1995) 'Capacity of minors to consent to medical and contraceptive treatment', *Medico-Legal Journal of Ireland,* Vol. 1, pp. 18-21.

Donnelly, M. (2002) *Consent: Bridging the gap between doctor and patient.* Cork: Cork University Press.

Douglas, G. (1992) 'The Retreat from Gillick', *Modern Law Review*, Vol. 55, p. 569.

Faden, R. and Beauchamp, T. (1986) *History and Theory of Informed Consent.* Oxford and New York: Oxford University Press.

Fallowfield, L.J., Hall, A., Maguire, G.P. and Baum, M. (1990) 'Psychological outcomes of different treatment policies in women with early breast cancer outside a clinical trial', *British Medical Journal,* Vol. 301, p. 575.

Faulkner, A., O'Keefe, C. and Peace, G. (1995) *When a child has cancer.* London: Chapman & Hall.

Fox, M. and McHale, J. (1997) 'In Whose Best Interests?', *Modern Law Review,* Vol. 60, p. 700.

Gabe, J., Olumide, G. and Bury, M. (2004) ' "It takes three to tango": A framework for understanding patient partnership in paediatric clinics', *Social Science & Medicine,* No. 59, pp. 1071-79.

Glasper, E.A. and Ireland, L. (eds) (2000) *Evidence-based child health care: Challenges for practice.* Basingstoke: Palgrave Macmillan.

Grubb, A. and Kennedy, I. (2000) *Medical Law Text and Materials,* 3rd edition. London: Butterworths.

Hammarberg, T. (1990) 'The UN Convention on the Rights of the Child – and how to make it work', *Human Rights Quarterly,* Vol. 12, p. 97.

Hanafin, S. and Brooks, A.M. (2005) *The Delphi Technique: A methodology to support the development of a national set of child well-being indicators,* National Children's Office. Dublin: The Stationery Office.

Hart, R.A. (1992) 'Children's Participation: From tokenism to citizenship', *Innocenti Essays,* No. 4. Florence: UNICEF Innocenti Research Centre.

Hill, M., Davis, J., Prout, A. and Tisdall, K. (2004) 'Moving the Participation Agenda Forward', *Children and Society,* Vol. 18, pp. 77-96.

Hill, M., Laybourn, A. and Borland, M. (1996) 'Engaging with primary-aged children about their emotions and well-being: Methodological considerations', *Children and Society,* Vol. 10, No. 2, pp. 129-45.

Hodgkin, R. and Newell, P. (2002) *Implementation Handbook for the Convention on the Rights of the Child.* Geneva: UNICEF.

Hogan, G. and Whyte, J. (2003) *JM Kelly: The Irish Constitution,* 4th edition. Dublin: Butterworths.

Irish Nursing Board (1988) *Code of Conduct.* Dublin: An Bord Altranais. Available at www.nursingboard.ie

John, M. (ed) (1996) *Children in charge: The child's right to a fair hearing.* London: Jessica Kingsley.

Kilkelly, U. (1998) 'In the Best Interest of the Child? An Evaluation of Ireland's performance before the UN Committee on the Rights of the Child', *Irish Law Times,* Vol. 19, pp. 293-300.

Kilkelly, U. (1999) *The Child and the ECHR.* Aldershot: Ashgate.

Kilkelly, U. (ed) (2004) *The ECHR and Irish Law.* Bristol: Jordans.

Kilkelly, U. and Lundy, L. (2006) 'Children's Rights in Action: Using the Convention on the Rights of the Child as an auditing tool', *Child and Family Law Quarterly* (forthcoming).

Kilkelly, U., Kilpatrick, R., Lundy, L., Moore, L. and Scraton, P. (2005) *Children's Rights in Northern Ireland.* Belfast: Northern Ireland Commissioner for Children and Young People.

King, N.M. and Cross, A.W. (1989) 'Children as decision-makers: Guidelines for paediatricians', *Journal of Paediatrics,* Vol. 115, No. 1, pp. 10-16.

Knafl, K.A., Cavallari, K.A. and Dixon, D.M. (1988) *Pediatric hospitalization: Family and nurse perspectives.* Illinois: Scott, Foresman & Co.

Lansdown, G. (2001) 'Promoting children's participation in democratic decision-making', *Innocenti Insight,* No. 6. Florence: UNICEF Innocenti Research Centre.

Law Reform Committee (2006) *Rights-based Child Law: The case for reform.* Dublin: Law Society.

Lowe, N. and Juss, S. (1993) 'Medical Treatment — Pragmatism and the search for principle', *Modern Law Review,* Vol. 56, p. 865.

Madden, D. (2002) *Medicine, Law and Ethics.* Dublin: Butterworths.

Maguire, P. and Pitceathly, C. (2002) 'Key communication skills and how to acquire them', *British Medical Journal,* Vol. 325, pp. 697-700.

Martin, F. (2004) 'The Ombudsman for Children: An analysis of the strengths and weaknesses of the Irish model', *Administration,* Vol. 52, No. 1, pp. 46-68.

McAuley, K. and Brattman, M. (2002) *Hearing Young Voices: Consulting children and young people, including those experiencing poverty or other forms of social exclusion, in relation to public policy development in Ireland.* Dublin: Open your Eyes to Poverty Initiative.

McGoldrick, D. (1991) 'The United Nations Convention on the Rights of the Child', *International Journal of Law and the Family,* Vol. 5, pp. 132-69.

McNeish, D. and Newman, T. (2002) 'Involving children and young people in decision-making', in *What works for children? Effective services for children and families,* D. McNeish, T. Newman and H. Roberts (eds). Buckingham: Open University Press.

Medical Council of Ireland (2001) *Review of Medical Schools in Ireland 2001.* Dublin: Medical Council of Ireland. Available at www.medicalcouncil.ie

Medical Council of Ireland (2004a) *Review of Medical Schools in Ireland 2003.* Dublin: Medical Council of Ireland. Available at www.medicalcouncil.ie

Medical Council of Ireland (2004b) *A Guide to Ethical Conduct and Behaviour,* 6th edition. Dublin: Medical Council of Ireland. Available at www.medicalcouncil.ie

Morgan, D. (2000) *Issues in Medical Law and Ethics.* London: Cavendish Publishing.

NCO (2000) *Report of the Public Consultation for the National Children's Strategy,* National Children's Office. Dublin: The Stationery Office.

NCO (2004) *Ready, Steady, Play! A National Play Policy,* National Children's Office. Dublin: The Stationery Office.

NCO, Children's Rights Alliance and National Youth Council of Ireland (2005) *Young Voices: Guidelines on how to involve children and young people in your work.* Dublin: The Stationery Office.

NYCI (2001) *Taking the Initiative: The involvement of young people in decision-making in the Republic of Ireland.* Dublin: National Youth Council of Ireland. Available at www.carnegieuktrust.org.uk

Phillips, J. and Grahn-Farley, M. (2002) 'International Child Rights at Home and Abroad: A Symposium on the UN Convention on the Rights of the Child. IV. Children's Rights to Health Care and Participation: United States Implementation of the UN Convention on the Rights of the Child', *Capital University Law Review,* Vol. 693, No. 30, pp. 700-01.

Pittman, K. (1992) 'Awakening child consumerism in health care', *Paediatric Nursing,* Vol. 18, No. 2, pp. 132-36.

Pridmore, P. and Lansdown, G. (1997) 'Exploring Children's Perceptions of Health: Does drawing really break down barriers?', *Health Education Journal,* Vol. 56, pp. 219-30.